"I love *I Am Not Alone* because it provides . Through her questions, Martha creates a platform for family caregivers to share the truth of their days, which empowers the reader to feel okay about their truths. I recommend this book for anyone impacted by FTD, anyone who works with family caregivers and every health care professional who interacts with a family managing an FTD diagnosis. This insightful book will leave you touched by the book's good company."

Denise M. Brown
CareGiving.com

"One of the biggest challenges to providing care for a person afflicted with dementia is the ever-increasing loneliness. As the illness progresses, the person with dementia slowly withdraws from conversations, activities, and social events leaving the caregiver isolated and virtually alone.

Many caregivers have limited access to others who can answer questions and provide moral support. Friends drop away. *I Am Not Alone* is a unique book of advice and encouragement offered by caregivers of people with dementia. It offers a realistic perspective developed to help caregivers feel less alone.

I Am Not Alone is essential reading for the family coping with dementia."

Geri R. Hall, PhD, CNS, FAAN

"Martha shines a light on a radically underexplored topic in most churches, in the medical community, and in our world: the lives of caregivers. Want to get better at caring for caregivers? Start here, by spending time with their stories, their joys and sorrows, hopes and fears. Learn what not to say and what's actually helpful. In so reading, you'll become a better friend."

Rev. Karl Fay
Prince of Peace Lutheran Church
Palatine, Illinois

I Am Not Alone

*Conversations with Care Partners of
People with Dementia*

MARTHA L. GARMON

Copyright © 2018 Martha L. Garmon
All rights reserved.
ISBN-13: 9781726892414

DEDICATION

To
Stephan
my love, my inspiration, my soulmate
you have been the love of Christ in my life
and have made me into the person
who could walk this road with you

Table of Contents

INTRODUCTION 1

ABBREVIATIONS 3

DEFINITIONS 5

MARTHA - Palatine, IL 9

SHARON - Cumming, GA 15

MARY – Roebuck, SC 19

TERRI – Minneapolis, MN 23

MARCIA – Ann Arbor, MI 27

GLENIS – Benton, AR 33

JULANE – Razorback, Australia 37

ANONYMOUS – NJ 43

ANNE – Tasmania, Australia 47

LORETTA – Arlington, MA 51

ANONYMOUS - WA 55

LORI – Skaneateles, NY 59

SHARON – Corfu, NY 63

DENISE – Thibodaux, LA 67

DANA – Indian Rocks Beach, FL 71

JIM – Barrington, IL 77

KIRSTIN – New Hartford, NY 81

MAJA – Moncks Corner, SC 87

MAUREEN – Seaford, DE 91

ANITA – North Royalton, OH 97

DEBBIE – Hornell, NY 103

LAURA – Carlisle, MA 109

LINDA – Tempe, AZ	113
RITA – Livingston, WI	117
CHRIS – Rio Grande, NJ	121
LEE – Discovery Bay, CA	125
SHELLI – Bakersfield, CA	131
KATHY – Hiawatha, IA	135
VICTORIA – Benson, NC	139
ANONYMOUS – United Kingdom	143
MAGGIE – South Wales, UK	147
TAMMY – Plymouth, IL	151
LINDA – Lexington, KY	155
ANONYMOUS - WA	159
GINA – Orrstown, PA	165
STEPHANIE – Dalton, MA	169
MARY – Two Rivers, WI	173
ELAINE – Federal Way, WA	177
ANONYMOUS - Canada	181
ANONYMOUS - KS	185
KATHY – Greenville, NC	189
NANCY – Eagan, MN	193
MY STORY	199
ACKNOWLEDGMENTS	205
APPENDIX 1: SUGGESTED READING	207
APPENDIX 2: RESOURCES	209
ABOUT THE AUTHOR	211

INTRODUCTION

Sometimes as care partners we feel very isolated and alone, especially when dealing with a disease as misunderstood as dementia. It feels like no one else can understand what we are going through. Well-meaning friends try to help by spouting platitudes or giving advice and end up making us feel worse and even more alone.

The good news is that we are not alone – there are others who know our struggle. The care partners who were interviewed for this book were asked to share what gives them hope. For some that was faith, for others support from friends or family. Regardless, I hope that you will find something in these interviews that will encourage you.

I wrote this book so that caregivers might find encouragement in reading about other's journeys, however, another use for this book is to give it to persons who are trying to support caregivers; so that they might have a better understanding of what we are feeling and/or needing from our support circle.

I have used the terms caregiver and care partner interchangeably. Some prefer the former, others the latter. Either way the journey is the same.

There are blank pages between some of the interviews, leaving space so you have room to make notes or to journal. There is a blank interview form at the end of the book so you can answer the questions for yourself, adding your voice to the conversation.

Most of the care partners interviewed here are married to persons who were diagnosed with frontotemporal degeneration (FTD). Many are part of the Facebook group for FTD Spouses. As for me, I don't know what I would do without these caregivers. Their combined knowledge and encouragement have been invaluable as I have walked this journey. The vast majority of care partners interviewed are women.

The statistics show that many women are also stricken with this disease, leaving their husbands as caregiver. Unfortunately, many of these male caregivers do not reach out for support.

Each of the participants in this project was presented with a list of twenty-three questions. I did my best to perform minimal editing to their answers, as I wanted their voice to be heard in their own way. One of the rules of the FTD Spouse group on Facebook is "no judgment." I hope that you can keep that in mind as you read the answers. Many of the answers may seem harsh, but I asked for honesty, and I applaud these care partners for sharing their honest feelings.

A few of the participants were widowed shortly before answering the questions. I'm sure, by the time of publication, more will have been widowed.

Some have chosen to remain anonymous and others have chosen to share their names. I am grateful to all who were willing to share their tears, their fears, the good, the bad, and their hearts.

Each participant gave their answers before they were allowed to see any of the other interviews. As you read, you will see there is a common thread in many of the interviews. As I stated earlier, at one time or another, we all feel isolated and alone. There is nothing we can do to change that completely, but I hope that by telling our stories and sharing our journeys, we might, just for a moment, realize that we are not truly alone.

Martha L. Garmon
Wife of Stephan, diagnosed FTD, July 2016; and ALS, February 2018

ABBREVIATIONS

ADL – activity of daily living, e.g. bathing, dressing, toileting, etc.
AFTD – The Association for Frontotemporal Degeneration
ALS – amyotrophic lateral sclerosis – also known as Lou Gehrig's disease
bvFTD – behavioral variant frontotemporal degeneration
FB - Facebook
FTD – frontotemporal degeneration
MND – motor neuron disease
GP – general practitioner
LO – loved one
MRI – magnetic resonance imaging
POA – power of attorney
PPA – primary progressive aphasia
PSP – progressive supranuclear palsy
TBI – traumatic brain injury
UCSF – University of California San Francisco
VA – Veteran's Administration

DEFINITIONS

Alzheimer's Disease (AD) is a type of dementia that causes problems with memory, thinking, and behavior. Symptoms usually develop slowly and get worse over time, becoming severe enough to interfere with daily tasks. (Alzheimer's Association – alz.org)

Frontotemporal degeneration (FTD) is a disease process that results in progressive damage to the temporal and/or frontal lobes of the brain. It causes a group of brain disorders that share many clinical features. FTD is also commonly referred to as frontotemporal dementia, frontotemporal lobar degeneration (FTLD), or Picks disease.

FTD is distinct from other forms of dementia in two important ways: First, the hallmark of FTD is a gradual, progressive decline in behavior and/or language (with memory usually relatively preserved). As the disease progresses, it becomes increasingly difficult for people to plan or organize activities, behave appropriately in social or work settings, interact with others, and care for oneself, resulting in increasing dependency on caregivers. Second, the onset of FTD often occurs in a person's 50s and 60s but has been seen as early as 21 and as late as 80 years. (Association for Frontotemporal Degeneration - theaftd.org)

Behavioral variant frontotemporal degeneration (bvFTD) is the form of frontotemporal degeneration (FTD) characterized by early and progressive changes in personality, emotional blunting, and/or loss of empathy. Patients experience difficulty in modulating behavior, and this often results in socially inappropriate responses or activities. Impairment of language may also occur after behavioral changes have become notable. (Association for Frontotemporal Degeneration - theaftd.org)

Motor neuron disease (MND) is a deterioration of motor neurons that manifest as weakness in the muscles with stiffness, difficulty making fine movements, atrophy (shrinkage) of the muscles, and fine muscle twitches and cramps. Muscle changes can affect the arms and/or legs on one or both sides of the body, or the face, tongue, and mouth, depending on how the nervous system is affected in that individual. (Association for Frontotemporal Degeneration - theaftd.org)

Amyotrophic Lateral Sclerosis (ALS) is a progressive neurodegenerative disease that affects nerve cells in the brain and the spinal cord. Motor neurons reach from the brain to the spinal cord and from the spinal cord to the muscles throughout the body. The progressive degeneration of the motor neurons in ALS eventually leads to the patient's death. When the motor neurons die, the ability of the brain to initiate and control muscle movement is lost. (ALS Association – alsa.org)

Primary progressive aphasia (PPA) is a language disorder that involves changes in the ability to speak, read, write, and understand what others are saying. (Association for Frontotemporal Degeneration - theaftd.org)

Progressive supranuclear palsy (PSP) is a rare brain disorder that causes serious and permanent problems with control of gait and balance. The hallmark of PSP is a visual disturbance, which results from a progressive inability to coordinate eye movements. PSP is related to both Parkinson's disease and FTD. (Association for Frontotemporal Degeneration - theaftd.org)

Semantic primary progressive aphasia (svPPA) is characterized by the progressive loss of the meanings of words. If there are additional major problems in identifying objects or faces, the condition is also called semantic dementia. Other language skills, including the ability to produce speech and to repeat phrases and sentences spoken by others, are unaffected. However, although the affected person may continue

to speak fluently, their speech becomes vague and difficult to understand because many words are omitted or substituted.
(Association for Frontotemporal Degeneration – theaftd.org)

Stephen Ministers are laypeople—Christian men and women—trained to provide one-to-one care to people experiencing a difficult time in life, such as grief, divorce, job loss, chronic or terminal illness, relocation, or separation due to military deployment. (Stephen Ministries - www.stephenministries.org)

MARTHA
Palatine, IL

"I pick myself up and keep going."

Caree and age at diagnosis: Stephan, 62
Diagnosis: FTD, July 2016; FTD/ALS, February 2018

Where do you find hope? Comfort? I find my hope and comfort in Scripture. My favorite Scripture is Revelation 21:4, "He will wipe every tear from their eyes. There will be no more death or mourning or crying or pain, for the old order of things has passed away." I know I will see Stephan again and he will be healed. This is my hope.

What is one thing about caregiving (or you or others) that surprised you most? I am surprised at how patient I can be with him. I am not a patient person. That is not to say that I am always patient, but in general I am better with him than I ever hoped I could be. A close second would be how many people think all dementias are the same. FTD is not Alzheimer's; and memory is not the primary function that is affected.

How do you take care of yourself? I have a Stephen Minister. I also try to make time to go out with friends when possible. At this point, I can still leave him alone for a couple of hours. I'm not sure what I will do when that is no longer possible. I also ask for help. That isn't easy for me, but I'm finding it to be necessary for my sanity. I also blog on Scripture to remind me from where my strength comes.

What do you do when you hit bottom? I have a good cry. Sometimes that means getting in the car and going around the corner, so I can be alone. After a good cry, I pray, then I pick myself up and keep going. I don't really have any other option; Stephan needs me.

What is the best/worst piece of advice you have ever been given? The best piece of advice was to get all our financial matters in order immediately after diagnosis. Knowing that everything is in my name and I have power of attorney over his matters has made everything so much easier. The worst piece of advice is when people come to me with articles telling me how eating this or that, or how using this device will make the dementia go away. We are registered in a database of available participants for clinical trials. If there was any hope out there, we would know about it. Herbal tea is not going to bring back the dead brain cells.

What is the best/worst thing you have learned about yourself? The best thing I have learned about myself is that I can be patient with Stephan. The worst thing I have learned is that I can't turn off my mind. It is constantly working not only on my to-do list, but on

Stephan's to-do list, the next appointment, making sure that financial matters are covered, getting the roof fixed, getting the snow shoveled, communicating with doctors re: symptoms, disease progression, appointments, payment, insurance...

What would you most like to tell someone who has become a caregiver? You will cry more than you ever thought possible. That's ok, don't be afraid to cry.

Another thing is to not make promises you can't keep. Instead of telling my husband that I'll never put him in a memory care unit, I say that I won't place him unless absolutely necessary. Small change in wording, but it keeps me from ever having to break a promise.

What would you do if someone handed you $100,000? Tithe to the church, then convert our bridge loan to permanent financing. Then when the old house sells, I would put the money in the bank to make sure I can pay whatever expenses come along for Stephan's care.

What would you do with three extra hours a day? I don't know. I know I should say exercise or take a bath, but I would probably try to get more of my list done.

What do you wish you had more of? People that I could call to help around the house.

What are some easy things you do to relax or find joy? Take a bath, dance to music, sew, watch a funny movie.

What is the best/worst question you have ever been asked? The best question would be "How are you doing?" from someone who really wants to know. The worst question was from a researcher, "Do you find purpose in your role as a caregiver?" No, I don't find purpose in that role. I don't want to be Stephan's caregiver, I want to be his wife.

What are three things someone could do to help YOU (not your loved one, but you)? Pick me up and take me out for a mani/pedi. Bring dinner over with a bottle of wine. Ask how I'M doing, not just Stephan, and then be willing to listen. Take Stephan for a weekend so I could go out without worrying about him.

When was the last time you cried? Today and most every day.

Do you like yourself? Yes, most of the time, but when I lose it with Stephan, then I don't.

What is the hardest thing you have faced? The thought of being a widow.

What is the one thing that no one can understand about your situation? How much it hurts to lose my best friend and all the dreams of our future together.

What is it that everyone should know, but no one wants to talk about? That my life changed on July 1, 2016. No matter how I wish it was not the case, there will always be a part of me that will be sad. Even on our best day, the disease will be looming in the background. Even if you don't want to talk about it, I am still thinking about it. My life, my heart, my everything, changed in just a moment.

Do you have support from family? Friends? Church? Others? Yes, mercifully, we are very blessed. His brother and sister-in-law are wonderful. Unfortunately, they are in another state, but they call and text to see how we both are doing. They also allow us to come stay as often as we can, which gives me some help from being the only one with him. We also have a young friend who comes down about once a month and gets me out of the house and spends time with Stephan as well. We also have a care coordinator at our church who helps us find people to step in and help when we need it. Our small group at church is also a huge help. They help with transportation for things he wants to do, as well as provide emotional and tangible support. I have several friends who check in on me and how I'm doing. They give me the chance to be "normal" for just a little while, cry when I need to, and just give me a big hug.

What do you miss the most? My best friend and our future dreams.

Do you have a humorous story you would like to share? Our joke is that I hope that when the day comes that he doesn't know me, he will call me "the nice lady that takes care of him." More likely, because of my bossiness, I will be "the mean lady that takes care of him." That joke always brings a smile to his face.

Anything else you would like to add? The best thing to say to me is, "Yeah, that sucks!" Don't try to make it better, you can't. The words "at least" should NEVER be used with someone who is hurting, it negates their feelings. When I say, "I'm fine" I'm not really, I'm just afraid if I told you the truth, you would quit asking. Being a caregiver is a very lonely journey, don't forget us.

List any resources that you have found helpful in your journey.
Theaftd.org
CareGiving.com

Roadid.com
TSA Cares
The FTD Spouse on Facebook

SHARON
Cumming, GA

"Forgive yourself, you are doing the best you can."

Caree and age at diagnosis: Rod, 62; Mom, 90
Diagnosis: Rod – bvFTD, January 2016, and Mom – vascular dementia, 2011

Where do you find hope? Comfort? I find hope in advocating. It empowers me to know what is being done to help those living with dementia and their care partners. I find comfort in accepting what can't be changed and learning all I can about the disease.

What is one thing about caregiving (or you or others) that surprised you most? What surprised me most was that I needed to emotionally separate to be a better care partner and look at things as being part of the disease, not intentional.

How do you take care of yourself? Rod and Mom go to a day center twice a week. This gives me time to be quiet and think and work on projects.

What do you do when you hit bottom? I cry, then dry my tears, forgive myself, and move on.

What is the best/worst piece of advice you have ever been given? Best advice was, from Pauline Boss' *Loving Someone Who Has Dementia*, that we must separate emotionally. Worst advice, I am not sure, I tend to block out well-meaning people with awful advice.

What is the best/worst thing you have learned about yourself? The best thing I have learned about myself, is that I am very good at speaking out and influencing others for better care and services. The worst thing I have learned about myself is that I can be very tenacious and need to watch when I need to back off.

What would you most like to tell someone who has become a caregiver? Relax, this is a long journey and if you wear yourself out in the beginning, you will resent the future. Find time for yourself, it is not selfish, it is self-preservation.

What would you do if someone handed you $100,000? Hmmm, well that isn't enough to do anything grand, but I think I would set up a respite program for care partners to be able to enjoy a weekend at a B&B (bed and breakfast).

What would you do with three extra hours a day? Slow down, take a walk, have dinner with friends.

What do you wish you had more of? Energy and contacts that can make a difference.

What are some easy things you do to relax or find joy? Talk to young people, their outlook is so refreshing and honest. Listen to soft music with my ear phones on and meditate. Laugh, a lot, at anything funny. Watch funny YouTube videos. Open my sun roof on beautiful days and turn up the radio.

What is the best/worst question you have ever been asked? Best question: "What one thing would help you most?" Worst question: "How do you do it?"

What are three things someone could do to help YOU (not your loved one, but you)? Ask me to go out to lunch. Take Rod and/or Mom out to lunch. Call me and just talk.

When was the last time you cried? Earlier this week. It happens less, but it hits me at odd times.

Do you like yourself? Absolutely.

What is the hardest thing you have faced? That my husband has changed in ways that hurt me greatly before we had a diagnosis.

What is the one thing that no one can understand about your situation? That I struggle with the same things everyone else does. People tend to think I can handle anything; I am not that strong.

What is it that everyone should know, but no one wants to talk about? That behavior variant FTD can cause very disturbing behavior and people hate to hear some of the things that would help others identify it in their own family.

Do you have support from family? Friends? Church? Others? Family? Yes, my son and daughter-in-law, but not my brother. Friends? Yes, they listen to me whine now and then. Church? Yes, I have a Stephen Minister that helps a lot. Others? I have great neighbors.

What do you miss the most? Camping in our travel trailer and traveling with Rod.

Anything else you would like to add? Relax, you are human, you will have good days and bad days. Forgive yourself, you are doing the best you can. Learn all you can about the disease you are dealing with; knowledge is power.

List any resources that you have found helpful in your journey. Online support groups, in person support groups, day programs for the "twins", dipping my toe into advocacy and seeing the tsunami of people who value a care partner's perspective.

MARY
Roebuck, SC

"I miss being a wife..."

Caree and age at diagnosis: Charles, 63
Diagnosis: PPA-FTD, 2013

Where do you find hope? Comfort? I find comfort when my husband has a good day, or with family and friends.

What is one thing about caregiving (or you or others) that surprised you most? As a caregiver, my biggest surprise was the amount of effort it takes every day to care for my spouse in a way that gives him the best quality of life.

How do you take care of yourself? I try to stay active, eat right, and get plenty of sleep.

What do you do when you hit bottom? When I hit bottom, I will cry the whole day.

What is the best/worst piece of advice you have ever been given? Best advice given to me was "never argue with a dementia patient." Worst advice was "speech therapy would help." (It didn't.)

What is the best/worst thing you have learned about yourself? The best thing I've learned about myself would be that my mind and body will do what it has to. Worst thing I've learned about myself is that I get overly stressed when something doesn't go as planned.

What would you most like to tell someone who has become a caregiver? I would advise a new caregiver to live in the moment. Stay away from yesterday and tomorrow.

What would you do if someone handed you $100,000? If someone gave me $100,000, I would immediately put it in savings for care for my husband in the future. Fees for nursing homes are a very scary thing for me.

What would you do with three extra hours a day? If I had three extra hours a day, I would do lunch with a friend, paint, and go to a spa.

What do you wish you had more of? I wish I had more support from family and friends.

What are some easy things you do to relax or find joy? For relaxation, I love my alone time at night. Reading, painting, talking to a friend, catching up on chores.

What is the best/worst question you have ever been asked? The best and the worst question I've ever been asked is "How is your husband?"

What are three things someone could do to help YOU (not your loved one, but you)? Things that would help me would be having more family and friend time. Having enough money saved for future facility care (so that I don't worry). Having someone to do activities with my husband to give me some down time.

When was the last time you cried? Last time I cried was yesterday.

Do you like yourself? Yes, I do like myself.

What is the hardest thing you have faced? The hardest thing I've ever faced was being told my husband has dementia.

What is the one thing that no one can understand about your situation? No one knows the emotional toll it takes on a spouse to be their caregiver.

What is it that everyone should know, but no one wants to talk about? Everyone should know that the "end stage" of this disease will come, and I am going to need help!!!

Do you have support from family? Friends? Church? Others? I have some support from family and friends.

What do you miss the most? I miss being a wife…and all that comes with being a wife.

Do you have a humorous story you would like to share? On the funny side here is that my husband cannot communicate (due to PPA), but he still loves to talk to strangers. Every time I see him heading towards a stranger, I'm trying to chase him down to say, "No, don't talk to strangers!!!"

List any resources that you have found helpful in your journey. My resources have been our neurologist, Center for Aging, other caregivers, support groups, Google, YouTube.

TERRI
Minneapolis, MN

"Often we feel like we are invisible."

Caree and age at diagnosis: Al, 64
Diagnosis: FTD/PPA with Parkinson's, October 2012

Where do you find hope? Comfort? Sometimes I can't find hope or comfort. When it does come, it is usually from Scripture, prayer, or music.

What is one thing about caregiving (or you or others) that surprised you most? How much I could do and how much I could tolerate and still feel a deep love for my husband.

How do you take care of yourself? I tried to eat healthfully since I was no longer able to go to the YWCA for exercise. I kept up my doctor appointments as well as my chemotherapy and radiation. If I wasn't healthy, I couldn't take care of my husband.

What do you do when you hit bottom? I cried, I begged God for help and comfort. Then I got up and did what had to be done. I had a few very close friends who were always there for me and for Al.

What is the best/worst piece of advice you have ever been given? The best advice I got was to get my legal affairs in order and take one day at a time. The worst advice I got was - try memory games, try coconut oil, etc. I wish someone would have advised me to record my husband's voice and take some videos before he progressed.

What is the best/worst thing you have learned about yourself? The best thing I have learned is how much I really loved my husband. The worst thing I learned is how mean and ugly I can get when I'm feeling angry and hopeless.

What would you most like to tell someone who has become a caregiver? Know your limits. Know that what is right for one person may not be right for you. If the patient is your loved one, you know better than anyone else what they need. Also, make memories while you still can and try not to be surprised when there is a decline. This is a progressive disease.

What would you do if someone handed you $100,000? At this point, I would donate it to theaftd.org to try to find a cure for this bastard disease.

What would you do with three extra hours a day? When I was a caregiver, probably exercise, read, or sleep. Now, I don't want three extra hours a day.

What do you wish you had more of? Time with my husband.

What are some easy things you do to relax or find joy? Deep breathing, listen to music, pray, read, walk.

What is the best/worst question you have ever been asked? Best – "Can I sit with Al, so you can get some time by yourself?" Worst – "Are you sure he isn't getting better? He looks terrific."

What are three things someone could do to help YOU (not your loved one, but you)? Try not to be uncomfortable when I cry. Go to a movie or a meal with me. I've gone almost five years without speaking to anyone because my husband was mute. Sit and talk with me.

When was the last time you cried? This morning (or now, if that counts).

Do you like yourself? Sometimes, other times not so much. The day before my husband died, I spent a lot of time telling him what a great husband and dad he was and apologizing to him for all the times I was mean and nasty to him because I felt so helpless. I'm still working on forgiving myself.

What is the hardest thing you have faced? Coming home to a dark, empty house after he passed away.

What is the one thing that no one can understand about your situation? How conflicted I am with my feelings, want to move on but can't let go, want to be happy but am always sad.

What is it that everyone should know, but no one wants to talk about? What that loss physically feels like after being "needed" 24/7 for such a long time. You really can feel your heart break.

Do you have support from family? Friends? Church? Others? I have three grown children, all who support in their own way. The last six months of Al's life, our oldest daughter was here every morning and evening (with some help from the other two) to help get him up or to bed. It's the only way I was able to keep him at home. I had help from Fairview Hospice and Tamarisk with respite workers. My church community was there, and close friends looked after both of us. A neighbor cut our grass every summer. I had a lot of support and still often felt alone because no one, and I mean no one, can walk in my shoes.

What do you miss the most? A healthy, happy husband, his laugh and his great hugs. I miss him saying "I love you" each night before I go to bed.

Anything else you would like to add? Thank you for thinking of the caregivers. Often, we feel like we are invisible, even to our loved ones because of the changes this disease causes.

List any resources that you have found helpful in your journey.
No Saints Around Here by Susan Allen Toth
Loving Someone Who Has Dementia by Pauline Boss
One Year Book of Hope by Nancy Guthrie
The Book of Psalms

MARCIA
Ann Arbor, MI

"Reach out – go against the instinct to isolate…"

Caree and age at diagnosis: Tom, 62
Diagnosis: FTD, July 2014

Where do you find hope? Comfort? I find comfort in savoring the simplest things of life – a warm fire, a beautiful sunset, time with family and friends. For me, hope is found in believing this is meant to be part of my life journey, that it is both meaningful and sacred. I also find comfort and hope in reflecting on things my ancestors went through, knowing that they had resilience and courage for it all, and hoping that will be my legacy as well. And, other care partners give me hope, as I watch their examples. They so frequently inspire me.

What is one thing about caregiving (or you or others) that surprised you most? Honestly, it has surprised me that I have been able to cope far better than I expected. I went through a severe mental health crisis just before my husband's diagnosis, and in the process received good professional care and a support system. I now have a coping "toolbox" that keeps me stable and at peace more consistently.

How do you take care of yourself? I participate in an online support chat twice a week and see a therapist. I try to make time for things I enjoy and also opportunities to pamper myself, even a simple foot soak before my husband wakes up in the morning. I do lots of mindfulness practices and try to make gratitude an active practice in my life. I find that gratitude is the best antidote for anxiety and depression for me. I ask myself, "Speaking as your own best friend, what do you need right now? A snack? A nap? A walk?" I'm smiling, because those are the questions you ask a child when they are in distress.

What do you do when you hit bottom? Reach out – go against the instinct to isolate or keep it secret that I'm having a difficult time. Call a trusted friend, see my therapist. I also find breathing and other meditative practices really help. It's easy to forget to breathe.

What is the best/worst piece of advice you have ever been given? Best: "Don't get ahead of the disease." It's easy to try to look into the future and cope with what is there. But there is no way to dress rehearse it. It must be lived moment by moment with what is happening in the present. I try to prepare (research, etc.) possible future decisions, but try not to live as though the future is happening already.

Worst: Before the diagnosis, I was told by some close friends that this was all my anxiety speaking; that I was overreacting. They also told me I needed to "honor my husband and go along with him." Worst advice ever. A true-blue friend was there to say, "Something is terribly wrong. Keep pursuing answers."

What is the best/worst thing you have learned about yourself? Best: I have learned that I am far stronger and more resilient than I would have ever known. Worst: I can sometimes really sweat the small stuff and need to be reminded of the big picture.

What would you most like to tell someone who has become a caregiver? First, you are not alone! In some form, most people are caregivers at some point in their life. Being a parent, being a child, being a friend. We all give care, this is just one way that a caring heart is expressed. And second, do not try to do it alone! This is more than one person can do. Assemble a strong team around you. Professionals such as lawyer and financial planner, community resources, friends and family, people to assist you with respite, people to help with repairs. Step by step, keep adding people to your team. Think of them as your teammates who will help you meet this challenge. A life coach suggested I replace the sentence, "I don't know how to…" with "I am in the process of, and I can't wait to see…" That was so helpful! I am in the process of assembling my team of helpers, and I can't wait to see who will be a help and encouragement to me.

What would you do if someone handed you $100,000? I'm not honestly sure. I hope that I would find a way to encourage other people with it. Providing respite for caregivers would be high on my list.

What would you do with three extra hours a day? Read, watch a movie, learn a new skill such as a second language.

What do you wish you had more of? Wisdom. Creativity for solving some of the practical problems. Mechanical skill for things around the house.

What are some easy things you do to relax or find joy? 1. Breathe. In, out, in, out. 2. Watch YouTube videos with either cute things like squirrel antics, or creative household hacks. 3. Read/watch things about spirituality and about hope. I love books and movies about true life, inspiring people who endured hardship and rose to meet challenges. 4. Soak my feet (water, vinegar, and mouthwash is incredibly refreshing.) 5. Talk heart-to-heart with a friend. 6. Send a card to someone you sense is lonely; anyone elderly you know is a likely candidate. 7. Smile. The physical act of gently smiling can actually change how my body feels.

What is the best/worst question you have ever been asked? Best: "What can I do to make this easier for you?" That made me cry, and I wanted to file it away to ask every single person in any kind of difficulty. Worst: "Let me know if you need anything." These two questions were likely posed by people who had the very best intentions. It's just that one put the responsibility on them, and one put the responsibility on me. It made a big difference.

What are three things someone could do to help YOU (not your loved one, but you)? Continue to treat us as a couple, ask us to do things that we can do. We can take a walk, sit in a park, watch a movie, listen to a concert. Don't stop inviting us. Offer to have my husband for an afternoon so I can do anything I want. Ask me what I need in the present – as in the friend who called to say, "I have several hours this afternoon. What do you most need me to do to help you?" A friend also showed up on my porch during our move to say, "Where would you like me to start?"

When was the last time you cried? Yesterday, dropping Tom off at his day program. I haven't ever cried about this before, but he looked particularly lost and forlorn. I got to the car and wept.

Do you like yourself? I think I actually do! I think I would like to have me as a friend, and I hope I am a good friend to myself as well as to others.

What is the hardest thing you have faced? Before the diagnosis, not knowing what was wrong, believing I was losing my marriage after 36 years. My husband was acting like someone I had never met. Absolutely terrifying and mystifying. Nothing made any sense. It was absolutely chaotic and crazy, and I couldn't get my bearings.

What is the one thing that no one can understand about your situation? I can't think of anything that no one can understand, because I have relationship with other care partners, and I believe they truly do understand. That is everything.

What is it that everyone should know, but no one wants to talk about? We are all mortal. Life is finite. Our loved ones are terminal, but so are we. My husband is dying. I am too. And neither of us knows the timing for either one of us.

Do you have support from family? Friends? Church? Others? I have a reasonable amount of support from family and friends. We made a 350-mile move to be in the same city with our child who lived the closest to us. My primary support system for being a care partner is the group of people I've met through online chat. We support one another in so many ways.

What do you miss the most? Going quickly to the store by myself to get a loaf of bread. Having a partner to care about me and how I'm doing. Being allowed to be the "not strong one" while my partner supports me. I now need to be the capable one 24/7. Going on errands by myself is a small detail, not having a full partner any longer is a huge loss. And yet they both make the list of "things I miss."

Anything else you would like to add? I learned from a friend that redwood trees have very shallow roots, and no tap root. They are actually held in place by all the other redwoods, which form a network of hair-like roots underground. We began calling one another redwoods, and the image of the redwoods brings me comfort and hope again and again.

Also, we will not do this perfectly. We are both learners and teachers through this journey. I have learned so much about life and love and what matters. And I believe I am also teaching, by example and by sharing with others. One way we teach is to teach others how to help us. Some truly want to learn.

List any resources that you have found helpful in your journey.
Several books have been indispensable to me:
Pauline Boss: *Loving Someone with Dementia* is like a guidebook to me.
Kristen Neff: *Self Compassion*
Lucy Hone: *Resilient Grieving*
Online support groups:
FTD chat on caregiving.com
FTD podcasts, same site
Teepa Snow videos
Mindfulness meditations (mindful.org has free resources you can receive every day)
Google it! Couldn't live without it. Everything from pureed food ideas to a video on how to change a person lying in bed. So many emotional/spiritual resources as well.
Mail order for all kinds of supplies (Amazon, etc.)
Grocery delivery services such as Shipt. Many grocery stores now also have "curbside pickup" which can be really handy when you can't be without your partner.

GLENIS
Benton, AR

"Give yourself grace…"

Caree and age at diagnosis: Allen, 66
Diagnosis: Alzheimer's and bvFTD, September 2016

Where do you find hope? Comfort? My faith in the Lord Jesus Christ is where I have my hope. I find comfort and hope in reading my Bible and praying.

What is one thing about caregiving (or you or others) that surprised you most? About caregiving – the emotional and mental strength it requires. I have to think of EVERYTHING now; how to care for him, how to manage his medications, how to keep him safe, how to run the household finances, how to keep the car running, how to buy big ticket items all by myself, how to handle difficult situations on my own.

How do you take care of yourself? I have learned to make sure I get enough sleep (that may change some day as he progresses). I try to make sure I enjoy my quiet time first thing in the morning. Also, eating better and taking my vitamins!

Another thing that helps me to cope on a daily basis is I have to simplify everything in my life. From literally cleaning and organizing my home, the paperwork for the running of the household, the grocery buying (our Walmart and Kroger have the ability to order online and you drive by to pick it up), the way I keep things tidy in the house (he can't tolerate anything out of place…it really works on the agitation if everything is in place).

What do you do when you hit bottom? I usually go to the bathroom and cry. If that is not an option, I will have to "run an errand" …get in the car, cry or literally scream. Then I pray; I pray a lot now.

What is the best/worst piece of advice you have ever been given? The best advice is that "If you have seen one person with dementia, you have seen one person with dementia." Every single person is different and will not be like the others. I can't expect him to act or progress like someone else.

What is the best/worst thing you have learned about yourself? How easily I can get angry at the least little thing; my lack of patience.

What would you most like to tell someone who has become a caregiver? Give yourself grace. You will make mistakes, you will make choices then you will second guess your decision but know that what you are doing is right for you and your loved one. There is no right way nor right answer. Follow your heart and do what you believe is right.

What would you do if someone handed you $100,000? Open an account in my name only (maybe with one of my adult kids on it) and put it in the bank to live off of when my husband passes.

What would you do with three extra hours a day? Go shopping, leisurely taking my time. I have to rush now so I can make sure I get home to him. Get a nice cup of coffee at Starbucks, just sit for a bit and listen to some favorite music uninterrupted.

What do you wish you had more of? Time with my husband before he became ill.

What are some easy things you do to relax or find joy? Play with my grandkids. Watch a favorite TV show. Sit out on the patio with a good cup of coffee. Pray to my heavenly Father as I watch my birdies in the yard.

What is the best/worst question you have ever been asked? "Is he going to get better?"

What are three things someone could do to help YOU (not your loved one, but you)? Come hang out with him while I run to get groceries. Talk with him and answer his questions that he repeats.

When was the last time you cried? I cry every day.

Do you like yourself? I'm on the fence about this…some days, I do like myself…other days, I see lots and lots of room for improvement.

What is the hardest thing you have faced? I think it was when my Mom passed away. She had Alzheimer's. And now my husband has FTD. This is just as difficult.

What is the one thing that no one can understand about your situation? The absolute loneliness that a spouse feels. I have no one to talk with about any of this or my feelings about dealing with FTD.

What is it that everyone should know, but no one wants to talk about? The guilt…the guilt of not doing enough, of hating this situation, the guilt of being angry with him, the guilt of wanting him to "go away" …it's the guilt of all those things.

Do you have support from family? Friends? Church? Others? I have minimal support from anyone.

What do you miss the most? The marriage relationship…not so much the physical part but the emotional connection…the little inside jokes. He has no deep caring or concern. The promise of what our lives would have been like in retirement...the dreams we had together...the security of him protecting me.

Do you have a humorous story you would like to share? I wish I did...that would help me as I can see the humor in situations, but he never did have a good sense of humor...so now, it's just sad for him.

Anything else you would like to add? I have learned to say "No" to anything that cause me extra work or would cause him added thinking or taking him out of his routine. It's all about his routine now. The holidays have wreaked havoc on him this year, such confusion.

You have to be in control of every aspect of your life. You have to dig deep within you to become a strong woman. You have to be slightly aggressive with doctors and nurses...establish a good relationship with your doctor's nurse (she/he conveys messages to the doctor).

You have to...it is a MUST...to put yourself first. Take care of you the best you can. Once I accepted his disease...and yes, it is a disease, my whole attitude changed. I wasn't so angry with him; I didn't blame him for the odd thinking, the weird behavior (he hasn't shown as many as some)! The frustration began to fade away from me once I accepted that he has a terminal brain disease...and that is what I tell people now.

JULANE
Razorback, Australia

"I treasure every moment we have together."

Caree and age at diagnosis: Jeff, 66
Diagnosis: bvFTD with suspected MND, September 2017

Where do you find hope? Comfort? Interestingly, my loved one first and foremost, as he has a reluctance to accept the diagnosis and so inspires me to continue my prayers for a miracle. But also, in our elderly dogs who give unconditional love and frequently catch my tears. And, spiritually, in my faith that keeps me praying for a miracle, but also gives me some comfort in the knowledge of the ever after.

What is one thing about caregiving (or you or others) that surprised you most? The serenity that come from finding something that works for my husband, especially when rewarded with a smile and the occasional heartfelt hug.

How do you take care of yourself? I have a small group of close friends with whom I regularly share updates on Jeff's condition, so I am not holding it in. I also actively volunteer as a firefighter and an international graded equestrian official; both communities give me amazing support and frequently assist with general maintenance around our property or odd jobs like errands, etc. I spend a little dedicated time every day with my horses and dogs for my own emotional welfare.

What do you do when you hit bottom? I cry, a lot! But then I either call our closest friend to download or go to church and pray for strength and guidance. I find openly talking to a close friend or my priest helps me cope just by not bottling up my emotions, fears, or frustrations.

What is the best/worst piece of advice you have ever been given? The best advice ever was to look after myself because if I fall over, my husband will have nobody to look after him.

The worst was to trust the medical professionals as I quickly came to realize their standard response was the generic option which was rarely the best for us. Once they realized I would not back down they completely changed their tune, worked out an individual care plan, and are working closely with me to make it succeed.

What is the best/worst thing you have learned about yourself? I never realized how strong I could be until I had to fight my husband's battles for him to make sure he received the best available care. I am pleased to find I have the inner fortitude to ensure he always gets the best result for what I know he'd have wanted when he was healthy.

The worst thing is that I sometimes pray this would all end as I struggle to see his suffering and know he'd never have wanted to live like this. And yet, I treasure every moment we have together and pray we may yet be in time for a miracle. And then I realize how selfish are those sentiments.

What would you most like to tell someone who has become a caregiver? Trust yourself, do what you believe is best first for yourself and then for your loved one and never give in to the establishment trying to make you decide something you don't feel is right for you. Find your inner strength and faith. And always remember, your loved one didn't choose this, has no control over what is happening to them, and cannot live up to your expectations so let them go – immediately!

What would you do if someone handed you $100,000? Firstly, I'd take the family on a last holiday together, probably to Disneyland as we always loved the park. And then I'd try to figure out if there was something, like equipment, that would help us keep my husband home for the long term that could eventually be handed onto someone without resources who would benefit from it. If there was more left over, I'd most likely give it to an FTD organization that provides aid to those in need.

What would you do with three extra hours a day? That's a trick question, as I fully retired when we got the diagnosis and so have all my time now at home looking after my husband. I don't currently sleep well and spend long hours when he is sleeping researching these diseases and looking for things that will either improve his day-to-day or will give me continued hope for our future. I should say I would catch a little more rest, but realistically, I would use the time to get more chores or more research/learning done.

What do you wish you had more of? Time. Metaphorically. I wish I knew we had more time so that we'd live long enough to beat this and continue our journey together into old age.

What are some easy things you do to relax or find joy? Cook. Being of Italian heritage I've always found cooking helps me to relax. Just chopping vegetables expends so many frustrations. Spend a few minutes petting or snuggling with our dogs; so much emotional strength derived from these guys. Take a walk around our property to commune a little with nature and breathe in fresh air. Sit out on the patio late at night and look up at the beautiful stars in the sky. Sneak out for an hour with one of the grandchildren and just soak up the simple joy of life through the eyes of a child.

What is the best/worst question you have ever been asked? The best – "What can I do to make it better for you?" When a friend genuinely asked how to help ease my burden and then followed through, it has taken away enormous stress from my daily life.

The worst – "Aren't you glad he was retired when it came on?" While the sentiment was right, the question cut me to the core. I wish with all my being it had never come on, period. But I do count my blessings daily for the full and happy life we have lived.

What are three things someone could do to help YOU (not your loved one, but you)? First, someone who could stay with him here at home one day each week, so I could get out, run errands, get groceries, meet a friend for a coffee, etc. That would give me peace of mind. Second, someone to do the basic chores outside that Jeff always did before, like mowing. That would give me pride in our home and time for other things. And lastly, someone to spend a week with me cleaning out closets and the shed, as so much has accumulated and it's difficult to motivate myself, but I know it would make me feel so much better were it all tidy and organized.

When was the last time you cried? Yesterday. Some days several times as I see my loved one's rapid decline. I normally cry 4-5 days each week at different triggers, but never in front of Jeff as I am desperate for him to retain hope for our future together.

Do you like yourself? Yes. I think I am an ok person who is devoted to my husband, our family, and our community.

What is the hardest thing you have faced? My husband's illness. I thought, when I lost my Granddad to cancer [when I was] 21, I would never experience such pain and suffering again. Then I lost Mum to the dreaded disease [when I was] 33. My in-laws lived with us and I was their primary carer, but by then I was a little hardened. But when my husband first fell ill, I was shattered, and every day a little piece of me is dying here beside him.

What is the one thing that no one can understand about your situation? My insistence to keep him home till death regardless how challenging his behaviors and the demands of caring for him. They don't understand my loyalty, as they think he is no longer the man to whom I pledged that loyalty. Even his children believe I should place him in residential care, as he's so difficult to manage day to day.

What is it that everyone should know, but no one wants to talk about? How the disease will progress and the worsening physical and mental condition that will impact us both.

Do you have support from family? Friends? Church? Others? I am truly blessed to have amazing emotional support on many levels. Some family members have been fantastic, but my husband's best friend has truly demonstrated unconditional friendship. He keeps our group of closest friends informed of events on a weekly basis, so people aren't making me relive everything over and over. I volunteer in the equestrian community and have had phenomenal support from people I know, including referrals to specialists and support services. We also are long-term volunteer firefighters and they have been amazing, offering counseling and support services and the boys doing odd maintenance jobs around our home for me. Our Brigade Minister checks on me every 2-3 weeks and gives me spiritual guidance, and my church gives me a great deal of spiritual support and inner strength. Compared to many, I am truly blessed.

What do you miss the most? The physical connection and my husband's wit. We used to be truly as one and always physically connected. Now he is often withdrawn and when we do hold hands or snuggle together, he is more detached. And, while there are still traces of his quick wit and sense of humor, he is much slower to process now and rarely enjoys a smile or a laugh.

Do you have a humorous story you would like to share? My husband has become obsessed with me, clearly with a deep underlying fear that I will leave him. So, as he started hiding things and becoming more possessive of me, I took our passports and hid them, so he couldn't hide them, or worse, destroy them. Do you think I have the vaguest idea where I've hidden them now?! Luckily there are no international trips planned in our immediate future.

Anything else you would like to add? FTD is an insidious disease, slowly robbing you of the person you know, but not in such a way for others to recognize and help. It took years to get a proper diagnosis and then several months to get all the necessary tests and treatment plan in place. Those were increasingly challenging times for both of us. His long-term GP doctor assumed we were having marital difficulties and ignored my pleas that something was seriously wrong; a peer whose spouse has PPA suffered exactly the same experience pre-diagnosis. The general community understands nothing of neurodegenerative diseases and lumps everything into the Alzheimer's category. There needs to be broader general education, as this is not a rare disorder and carers become so isolated and vulnerable due to ignorance.

The most challenging thing for me is my husband's inability to accept the disease and his lingering strong sense of pride. I cannot have anything mentioned in any public forum as he thinks people don't see he is ill, and I must preserve his pride, as that keeps him fighting. All of my research is clandestine, and so the internet is invaluable. In our case, my biggest single issue is my husband perceives this to be a mental disorder rather than physical; we must change that community perception for future generations. This is a disease, just like cancer, diabetes, or leukemia; we must get society to hear that message and change perceptions and expectations.

List any resources that you have found helpful in your journey.

There are many, so my first and best resource was Google. Google set me on a never-ending path of information about the disease. In fact, Google first told me what this was, as after husband's MRI, I came home and googled dementia, found the US organization, read about differing types, and as soon as I read bvFTD, I knew exactly what he was suffering, as he ticked every single box perfectly. I have learned so much through Google searches and then following the trails. And I have found specialist support which has helped me immensely.

For my own emotional support, I have found several Facebook closed groups exceptional. In my case, the FTD Spouse group has been by far the best, as members are experiencing similar things to me; they genuinely understand. The FTD support group has also been excellent, as there are numerous resources posted there.

I find the university sites especially helpful and think somehow the dementia organizations should tap into that depth to become the one-stop shop.

ANONYMOUS
New Jersey

"Take a deep breath!"

Caree and age at diagnosis: Spouse, 57
Diagnosis: Primary Progressive Aphasia

Where do you find hope? Comfort? Time with my three children (aged 22, 20, and 17) gives us joy and comfort. Only they can get close to understanding what I feel. Hope comes in my hoping they have a good future life in spite of what is happening to their dad.

What is one thing about caregiving (or you or others) that surprised you most? It is quite a roller coaster. You want to provide and care for your loved one, but you hate the disease and how it has changed them. Certainly, he is not the man I fell in love with 28 years ago. Yet when the smallest glimpse of the old "him" comes through, it just melts me.

How do you take care of yourself? Support group has been a life saver. I have formed friendships with people who can relate. I also try to plan monthly get-togethers with old friends, even if just for coffee or lunch.

What do you do when you hit bottom? I cry a lot. Mostly at night in my bed away from my son. Also, sometimes when I am visiting my husband. The tears usually come out of nowhere and hit me like a Mack truck. Uncontrollable! Very sad, but a bit cathartic, too.

What is the best/worst piece of advice you have ever been given? The best piece of advice was to put my children first! I met a man whose wife passed away in her late 40s from this. His children were around my children's age, and he told me to make time for the kids and me, and to get the kids away from it all so they can enjoy themselves and each other. The worst piece of advice came from my brother (who is a physician). He keeps bugging me to get my husband re-evaluated. We had gone for a second opinion when he was diagnosed four years ago. The neurologists we saw are at the University of Pennsylvania and Johns Hopkins, both top institutions. To try and get another evaluation now when my husband can hardly do any of the ADLs is absurd!

What is the best/worst thing you have learned about yourself? I learned how much I can handle. People always tell me how strong I am, and that God only gives you what you can handle. I think we can all handle what comes our way. We have to! Worst thing is that many times I am not really that strong. I don't want to deal with this or live through another day. But my husband and my kids still need me, so go on I must!

What would you most like to tell someone who has become a caregiver? Take a deep breath! Get help as soon as possible! Listen to experts! The director at an adult day center told me in plain words what was going to happen. Hard to hear, but necessary! Find a support group where you feel that you fit in and be yourself! Allow yourself to make mistakes, but don't feel guilty. We are navigating a mine field with no map and each of our carees is different! There is no right answer. Also appreciate the small miracles of every day: a knowing look, hand holding, a good day (or even a good hour) can all be miracles!

What would you do if someone handed you $100,000? Retrofit my house so I can have my husband come back and live there. I would need a room for a live-in caregiver and a first-floor full bath.

What would you do with three extra hours a day? Exercise, sleep, and chip away at the clutter in my house.

What do you wish you had more of? Time: time with my husband to just sit and hold hands, with my kids doing everything and nothing, time to travel and see my extended family who live abroad.

What are some easy things you do to relax or find joy? Watch a favorite show with one or more of my kids, listen to podcasts while I walk, read before bed, get together with friends, and sit with my husband.

What is the best/worst question you have ever been asked? Best question: "What have you been doing to take care of yourself?" Worst questions: "What have you been doing to take care of yourself?"

What are three things someone could do to help YOU (not your loved one, but you)? Take my son for a few days so I can go to a wedding. Visit my husband so I know he is not alone, and I can do something else without feeling guilty. I want my parents to go away this winter to visit our family abroad, so I don't have to worry about them in this cold weather.

When was the last time you cried? Four days ago.

Do you like yourself? Sometimes. I never had much patience and being a single parent to a teenage boy is bringing out the worst in me, especially when having to deal with FTD.

What is the hardest thing you have faced? Placing my husband! It has been six months and I still doubt that decision and try to think of ways to bring him back.

What is the one thing that no one can understand about your situation? Not only is caring difficult emotionally, physically, and financially, but absolutely losing my best friend is insane. Also, no one can understand that I pretty much cannot think of making any plans for the future, even if it is a few weeks away, let alone long-term plans! Most people have some kind of a vision of how they want their life to be. I am unable to have a future "vision/plan/fantasy". People tell me I am young (51 years old) and can still have a whole other life. But I am terrified. The thought of meeting someone else to start a new life is so scary. Partly because – what if that person develops dementia (or something else)?? Crazy right?! I cannot go through it again.

What is it that everyone should know, but no one wants to talk about? How when your spouse becomes incontinent, caregiving takes on a whole other meaning. Also, if they become violent/aggressive when they never were before. It just rocks you to your core.

Do you have support from family? Friends? Church? Others? Yes, I have the best parents and children. My husband's siblings are caring as well and visit him when they can. I have lots of friends from when I had a normal life and others I met in support groups.

What do you miss the most? Conversation! Having someone to talk to throughout the day and at the end of the day. A partner to share life with.

Do you have a humorous story you would like to share? Last time we went to the neurologist, my husband wouldn't sit still at all. He kept pacing and couldn't answer any questions the doctor asked him. At one point, he pointed to the doctor and said, "He's weird."

Anything else you would like to add? There is a lady who lives in my husband's facility. She is around his age (early 60s) and they hang around each other. Just sitting or walking mostly. But I am happy it brings them both comfort.

List any resources that you have found helpful in your journey. Theaftd.org website is full of information. The FTD Spouse and other Facebook closed groups are very helpful with hints and suggestions and knowing someone else is going through this.

ANNE
Tasmania, Australia

"Don't take anything personally."

Caree and age at diagnosis: Nick, 61
Diagnosis: bvFTD, 2013

Where do you find hope? Comfort? On-line support group, daughter, and grandchildren.

What is one thing about caregiving (or you or others) that surprised you most? The ignorance and misunderstanding of this disease by some family and friends.

How do you take care of yourself? I am currently waiting to see if I am eligible for a self-help group and also have Nick booked into four blocks of two-week respite for 2018.

What do you do when you hit bottom? Cry, cry, and cry some more.

What is the best/worst piece of advice you have ever been given? The best advice was when first diagnosed, our physical geriatrician told us to get all our financial affairs in order, get power of attorney and guardianship.

What is the best/worst thing you have learned about yourself? In the beginning, the worst thing I learned about myself was that I could feel so resentful.

What would you most like to tell someone who has become a caregiver? Get all the education you can, don't take anything personally, and when you can get a break, do so without feeling guilty.

What would you do if someone handed you $100,000? Help my family.

What would you do with three extra hours a day? Go insane…my days are spent trapped at home as my husband spends all his day in his room either sleeping or on his computer…he never wants to go anywhere or do anything, but he can't be left alone either.

What do you wish you had more of? Being included in family and friends' things.

What are some easy things you do to relax or find joy? My grandchildren, crochet, games on net, and reading.

What is the best/worst question you have ever been asked? Often asked how long I am going to keep caring for Nick before I put him into a permanent care home.

What are three things someone could do to help YOU (not your loved one, but you)? 1. Someone to come and take me fishing…I really miss that. 2. Someone to do some handyman jobs. 3. Sometimes, someone to just give me a big hug.

When was the last time you cried? Today at the doctor's.

Do you like yourself? Hard question…I feel like I have lost myself along the line somewhere. Don't really like or dislike myself.

What is the hardest thing you have faced? My husband being sexually inappropriate to our then thirteen-year-old granddaughter …fortunately, the sexual inappropriateness, porn, etc. stage seems to have passed, but that was hard to deal with. Also, he would have instant flashes of anger, so went through a very long period where I was actually, on occasions, a bit scared of him. But thanks to progression and meds, that seems to have also passed. Also, it was so terribly hard before diagnosis as you are trying to deal with things when completely in the dark as to why they were happening.

What is the one thing that no one can understand about your situation? No one sees the real situation, as he can still put up a good front when others are around. It's not like Alzheimer's'…his memory is still very good. He can "parrot" what he has been told, what's on the news, etc. and can still hold a conversation if he has to, but he can't make decisions, his logic and planning are affected; he has no empathy and deep apathy. Most people don't get that.

What is it that everyone should know, but no one wants to talk about? It is a terminal disease, no cure, and can take many years. But no matter how long it takes, it does progress, and you watch the person you love, who once was a high functioning person, change into someone so different and there is not a thing you can do to fix it…very cruel, more so for the families, I believe, as in our case. Nick is content (because of his apathy and meds) as long as he knows where I am, has his bed, food, and iPad; nothing else matters to him.

Do you have support from family? Friends? Church? Others? I have four daughters, but only one who is supportive, and she goes above and beyond. I have a wonderful brother who I can call on at any time, a lovely sister who lives a long way away, but will always listen, and a couple of friends who do call in when they can. Other family and friends have disappeared.

What do you miss the most? I miss my husband. Even though he is still here, he is not. I miss his quick sense of humor, I miss having him to talk with, make life decisions with, the life we had, the life we planned to have. I miss his hugs, his shoulder to lean on, but most of all, I miss his caring about me.

Do you have a humorous story you would like to share? Lots of funny things do happen, but you kind of have to be there at the time, and most of them, although funny, when I actually go to write them, they are also sad really, and I feel like I am mocking him or being disloyal to him in a way.

Anything else you would like to add? I hate this rotten disease.

LORETTA
Arlington, MA

"My brain never stops."

Caree and age at diagnosis: Tom, 62
Diagnosis: FTD, March 2015; PSP, September 2017

Where do you find hope? Comfort? I pray for some reason to Mary the most, and Saint Dunphna, the patron saint for neurological diseases. My adult children give me comfort.

What is one thing about caregiving (or you or others) that surprised you most? How emotionally draining it is, my brain never stops.

How do you take care of yourself? Probably not good enough, I used to walk with a friend, but I find it difficult now because that means leaving him alone.

What do you do when you hit bottom? Cry and pray, sometimes eat ice cream.

What is the best/worst piece of advice you have ever been given? Both best/worst – "You need to take care of you, you need time for yourself" …really? Best – "We have no control of this; none, however, we can control how we react to it; we need to keep on living."

What is the best/worst thing you have learned about yourself? Best: I am more compassionate for people with real problems. Worst: I have little tolerance for people that complain about little things. I know a woman who was going to Hawaii with her daughter, she complained about how tired she was going to be when she got there. Are you kidding me??!

What would you most like to tell someone who has become a caregiver? You can do it, it's hard, but you can do it. There are days it's just so worth it, when he looks at me and smiles, which isn't often, my heart melts. I would be honest and also tell them it hurts your heart.

What would you do if someone handed you $100,000? Take my whole family on a vacation to the ocean; as a family we always enjoyed the ocean.

What would you do with three extra hours a day? I honestly don't know. I don't sleep well, so that's out. I just don't know.

What do you wish you had more of? More time with my husband before this disease took him from me, then money to take better care of him.

What are some easy things you do to relax or find joy? I find joy in my new granddaughter, being with my kids, being alone, and taking a walk - this doesn't happen often anymore; it would mean leaving him alone.

What is the best/worst question you have ever been asked? Worst: "What are you doing for you?" Best: An older woman, whose husband passed from cancer several years ago told me, "At the end of the day, it's just you and him." She was right.

What are three things someone could do to help YOU (not your loved one, but you)? Visit with my husband. I know that's for him, but it makes my heart feel good to see that someone cares, so it's also for me. Send me a card, just telling me you care. Understand that I don't have the time I did to do things.

When was the last time you cried? Today.

Do you like yourself? Yes, most of the time.

What is the hardest thing you have faced? Watching the man I married become a shell of what he was. It breaks my heart. Also, seeing what it has done to my kids.

What is the one thing that no one can understand about your situation? The feeling of isolation.

What is it that everyone should know, but no one wants to talk about? He's already gone. He's breathing, but he's gone.

Do you have support from family? Friends? Church? Others? I have three adult children that help, but I hate to burden them; they are just starting their adult lives.

What do you miss the most? The love we had for each other. I know he loved me, and he can't anymore.

Do you have a humorous story you would like to share? About a year ago (he couldn't express this now) we left the neurologist's office and I took him to lunch. He looked at me and said, "You better take care of yourself. If your brain starts shrinking, we are going to be in deep sh**!"

Anything else you would like to add? Several years ago, I read the book *Tuesdays with Morrie*. Something I always remembered was when he was asked how he gets through this terrible disease, he replied (not exact words) that he allows himself fifteen minutes every day to cry and feel bad for himself and then gets on with living. I try to do that.

List any resources that you have found helpful in your journey. The booklet that the FTD foundation, not sure of the name, has for free. I ordered a bunch to give to the kids and my family/friends to read. The book, *What If It's Not Alzheimer's*. I joined, online, the FTD Spouse group.

ANONYMOUS
Washington

"I miss everything about being married."

Caree and age at diagnosis: Spouse, 49
Diagnosis: FTD, 2016

Where do you find hope? Comfort? I'm not sure I've found hope anywhere. I have found comfort in reading books about my situation, support groups (in person), online support groups, therapy sessions, being open with friends and family about my situation, and taking care of myself.

What is one thing about caregiving (or you or others) that surprised you most? I've been most surprised at how little support is given by friends or family. Perhaps they are waiting for a larger tragedy or perhaps they are in denial. I've also been shocked by the number of doctors that treated my situation as if I was the problem. The doctors don't want to take away hope, but in doing that they take away every opportunity for the caregiver/family to accept the diagnosis. It's enormously damaging.

How do you take care of yourself? I get out of the house by myself as much as possible. I attend two support groups monthly. I have a monthly massage appointment. I see a therapist every two weeks. I prioritize my needs/wants over my husband's. This is easy because he has no needs or wants, but it's taken me nearly a decade to come to terms with this.

What do you do when you hit bottom? Bottom is usually a lot of crying. The crying used to last literally hours, sometimes several days. I finally had to stop crying because it took so much out of me physically. When I reach bottom, I rest. I will get into bed. Have a cup of tea. Watch a movie. Usually I feel physically better in the morning. The emotional part never feels better. I also reach out to the online support groups because those are available 24/7 and give me a place to vent. Hearing from people who have experienced the same situations gives me a boost. It's good to know I will live through this.

What is the best/worst piece of advice you have ever been given? Worst advice, well there's so much! "Don't focus on it." "What if you split up and got him an apartment, wouldn't that help him?" "Treat the depression," has been said many times by doctors, but when I would ask what treatment they would recommend, they went silent.

Best advice, "You will live through this, he won't."

What is the best/worst thing you have learned about yourself? The best thing I have learned is that I'm resilient and confident. The worst thing is that I can be stuck for a very long time, like ten years, and I cannot get that time back.

What would you most like to tell someone who has become a caregiver? Put things in place to guarantee you can take care of yourself. Big things, if you can, like travel, or work. Small things, too. Protect your health. Sleep, eat, get checkups. You are important.

What would you do if someone handed you $100,000? I would take it as a sign that I should worry less about money! I might run for political office and fix the healthcare system. It's terrible that so many people are bankrupted by illness.

What would you do with three extra hours a day? I'm really not sure, but I would enjoy having that time.

What do you wish you had more of? Places to go and people to go with.

What are some easy things you do to relax or find joy? Watch movies, have a tea or coffee or cocoa, go out to eat, travel, and sew/quilt.

What is the best/worst question you have ever been asked? The best question I've been asked is whether I still have an intimate relationship with my husband. The question made me feel that my friend truly understood the depth of my loss.

The worst question is always… "Have you tried <insert exercise/vitamin/goal>?" This is so awful because our diagnosis took five years. Of course, we tried that! I'm not dumb.

What are three things someone could do to help YOU (not your loved one, but you)? I could use help finding a job so that I could be out of the house more. I feel like with the right job I can afford help at home and not have to take care of him at every stage myself.

When was the last time you cried? Two days ago. I'd probably be crying now, except that I'm in Starbucks and there's some happy music on.

Do you like yourself? Yes, I do. :)

What is the hardest thing you have faced? Losing my husband. He has rejected me over and over because his frontal lobe issues don't allow him to remember relationship stuff. Second hardest thing was getting a diagnosis.

What is the one thing that no one can understand about your situation? How he looks and acts so functional yet is qualified for disability. I'm not sure people believe he has FTD.

What is it that everyone should know, but no one wants to talk about? FTD is terminal. The timeline is uncertain. There will be a physical decline that likely includes incontinence, weight loss, inability to walk or speak. It's okay to ask about how the illness is affecting the family. We shouldn't be forced to hide from reality.

Do you have support from family? Friends? Church? Others? I get brief support when I provide friends and family with an update. No one reaches out, and I often feel they assume I am okay.

What do you miss the most? I miss everything about being married.

List any resources that you have found helpful in your journey.
FTD Spouse group on Facebook
TheAFTD.org to find an in-person support group
Book: *Green Vanilla Tea* (written by a woman with two teens whose husband had FTD)

LORI
Skaneateles, New York

"Learn to accept offers of help."

Caree and age at diagnosis: Thomas, 54
Diagnosis: ALS, 2007; FTD, 2008 (although I knew the FTD even sooner than the ALS); and Alzheimer's on autopsy…all three!

Where do you find hope? Comfort? Early on, I remember taking a moment (when alone feeding the cats), to sing the Good Morning song one sings to children. I would envision a future with grandchildren to love and cherish…I would sing to them. And now I have two!! With one more due soon.

How do you take care of yourself? I never stopped walking or running outside with friends. It took care of three things at once: fresh air, exercise, and talk therapy! When possible, I also went to one exercise class – often Pilates. It gave me quiet time and kept me in shape. I often cried during Pilates…a quiet cry no one else could see…the mind-body connection.

What do you do when you hit bottom? Write about my feelings. Call them out. Bring them into the air to breathe; then let them go.

What is the best/worst piece of advice you have ever been given? Early on someone told me, "This is a marathon, not a sprint. Take it day-by-day. Live in the now." Also, "Don't worry about what will come in the future…just focus on today and what you can handle." If I would have worried about what was to come, I would have been worrying about the wrong things anyway!

What is the best/worst thing you have learned about yourself? I learned I am stronger and more capable than I knew. I learned how deeply I loved Tom.

What would you most like to tell someone who has become a caregiver? Don't forget to take care of yourself. Everyone told me that. Sometimes I didn't know what they even meant. Also: Learn to accept offers of help. Say yes. This was hard…I was used to being the one who gave help. But sometimes we must receive help. It also helps others to be able to feel they can do something.

What would you do if someone handed you $100,000? If someone is a caregiver without help, they should use the $100,000 to get help. To have freedom, to gain time. This wasn't an issue for me because we were blessed with long term care insurance, so I had access to caregivers and thus I had freedom. I went to work every day and used caregivers to go on walks, etc. It made me a better caregiver and it saved my sanity.

What would you do with three extra hours a day? What would I have said to this? I never had enough time. At the time I might have said I would spend it in the fresh air, or seeing my family, or writing, or exercising, or sleeping!!! Now I would say I wish I would have spent it hugging Tom more. Dancing with him. Making his eyes sparkle.

What do you wish you had more of? Time. Always. In sickness and in health!

What are some easy things you do to relax or find joy? Walk in the fresh air. Swim in a lake. Run. Feel the air. (I can leave work feeling tired and depleted. I feel the air and I come alive.)

What is the best/worst question you have ever been asked? BEST questions were honest, probing ones. "What is this like for you?"

What are three things someone could do to help YOU (not your loved one, but you)? Ask and listen. Visit and offer to take him places for me. Random, welcome things like dropping off food, or cleaning my gutters! (Really! People did.)

When was the last time you cried? Yesterday.

Do you like yourself? Yes.

What is the hardest thing you have faced? Grappling with the fact that I lost hold of the real feel of the memories, the real Tom. And my son did too, and it is painful for him.

What is the one thing that no one can understand about your situation? The insidiousness of the loss. The way we never got to say goodbye. Here is something I wrote for the FTD site:

Nobody but us
knows what it is like to miss someone you love
while you sit with them, look at them, and help them through the day.
Nobody but us
knows the torment
the absolute splitting of yourself in two
that comes with being there, together and loving, on the one hand,
and being so far away on the other
that there is no connection in sight, ever again.
Nobody but us
knows what it is to try not to cry too soon;
to hold back tears, and memories, because the person you once loved
is still at your side.

In this life, we all lose people we love
we all miss people and grieve for people and long for people
and hold on to loved ones in our memories.
But, nobody but us knows the internal conflict
that comes with missing and longing and grieving
while the person you love is right next to you.

Do you have support from family? Friends? Church? Others? Yes. Living in a small community is helpful. Some of the people who have showed up are not who I would have imagined, and some of those I would have expected a bit more of (family far away, etc.) showed up less than I would have predicted. I think it is BEST not to judge. Don't spend time lamenting those who don't show up. Instead, celebrate those who do. Our house was always inviting. It was still a place people liked to be.

What do you miss the most? The real guy. His spirit. His strength. I miss how he stopped remembering our history, our stories, the things we knew, the two of us. I had to carry them without him.

Do you have a humorous story you would like to share? Yes. Love this one: A friend/caregiver was trying to get him into the house and he was refusing to use the ramp. He was standing at the steps, but we all knew he couldn't walk up steps. She finally said, "Why are you being so obstinate?" and he quipped back, "I am not being obstinate, I'm being an asshole." This was clear as a bell, something he once would have said...like he was coming back through a fog.

Anything else you would like to add? He always said, "It is what it is." Caregivers should remember that the obstinate behavior is not the real person. This is an illness. Don't point out the mistakes. Be loving and forgiving, and that will be calming.

List any resources that you have found helpful in your journey.
The book *Ambiguous Loss*
More than anything: communicating with people who were going through the same thing or had gone through it. I wish I had known about the FTD Facebook pages!!! Didn't learn of these until after his death.

SHARON
Corfu, NY

"Don't try to anticipate what is coming."

Caree and age at diagnosis: Mark, 55
Diagnosis: bvFTD, July 31, 2015

Where do you find hope? Comfort? I have a lot of faith in God and know that he is with me every step of the journey.

What is one thing about caregiving (or you or others) that surprised you most? When it is necessary, you can do whatever needs to be done, including installing doorbells and smoke detectors.

How do you take care of yourself? When hubby's needs are cared for, I go to my bedroom by myself and enjoy my dogs. I also get a massage once a month.

What do you do when you hit bottom? Cry and curse as needed, and then pick up the pieces and go on!

What is the best/worst piece of advice you have ever been given? The best advice what that it was ok to be angry, and although I care for his needs, don't consider myself his mother, but rather his coach. Worst advice was to contact his family for help. It just proved they didn't care about him and his situation and made me sad.

What is the best/worst thing you have learned about yourself? The best thing is also the worst thing. I am not a born caregiver. That realization has given me the strength to accept it and deal with situations in my own way.

What would you most like to tell someone who has become a caregiver? Don't try to anticipate what is coming. Each day has its own troubles.

What would you do if someone handed you $100,000? Place my husband in memory care and pay off his debt.

What would you do with three extra hours a day? Smell the roses…enjoy my home and grandchildren.

What do you wish you had more of? Money. This disease has taken everything I worked for, including prior to our marriage.

What are some easy things you do to relax or find joy? Watch crime shows, snuggle with my Boston terriers, take a hot bath, cook, visit with friends on text or Facebook.

What is the best/worst question you have ever been asked? Worst: "Is he getting better?" Best: "How are you doing and how can I help?"

What are three things someone could do to help YOU (not your loved one, but you)? Invite me to an afternoon out (when hubby is at daycare). Invite BOTH of us to dinner. Hubby still does well at restaurants. Come visit him so I can go out to do errands.

When was the last time you cried? Today…it is a daily occurrence.

Do you like yourself? I do…I hate how I am living, however.

What is the hardest thing you have faced? Dealing with the financial mess he created…especially with the IRS.

What is the one thing that no one can understand about your situation? Because he appears so "normal", people can't understand what it is like to grieve someone still living. The man I married is long gone, replaced by an angry stranger.

What is it that everyone should know, but no one wants to talk about? Neurodegenerative diseases are fatal; they are never going to get better; today is the best they will ever be.

Do you have support from family? Friends? Church? Others? A couple of MY childhood friends will still go out to dinner with us; my church family does not come to visit. I have no support from my family or my husband's family. I am pretty much on my own.

What do you miss the most? Traveling.

Do you have a humorous story you would like to share? For our twentieth wedding anniversary I sent myself flowers with his name on them. When they arrived, he asked who the flowers were from. I told him to read the card. He looked at it and said, "How did that happen?" Gave me a good chuckle.

List any resources that you have found helpful in your journey. The FTD Spouse group on Facebook has been my lifeline.

DENISE
Thibodaux, LA

"Now it just seems to be a waiting game."

Caree and age at diagnosis: David, 57
Diagnosis: FTD, March 2016 (symptoms since late 2012); MND, December 2017

Where do you find hope? Comfort? I find hope in my family, particularly my children and grandchildren. It is truly because I have their support and encouragement that I am able to get through each day. They assure me that a future does exist, albeit, not the future I envisioned.

What is one thing about caregiving (or you or others) that surprised you most? The most surprising thing about caregiving is the heavy feeling of isolation. Although my family visits and calls quite often, the time is spent mostly on the subject of David's illness. Some friends do visit or call periodically, but nothing compared to our interactions prior to his illness. One friend has actually told me that David's friends just do not want to see him this way. I do try to be understanding, but sometimes that is hard and only adds to the feeling of isolation.

How do you take care of yourself? I really have not done a good job of taking care of myself. I do walk periodically, but not as often as I could. One of the things I have noted in my Things to Do in 2018 is to schedule all of my appointments (doctors, dentist, eye, etc.). I have also begun the process of finding someone to stay with David once a week so that I can just do something fun. I would love to attend a yoga/meditation class and do a little self-pampering (spa day or mani/pedi). Hope to get that in place in February.

What do you do when you hit bottom? I call a friend. I have one good friend that is always there to just listen. Applies no judgment and most times doesn't even need to provide advice, as I often know the answer but just need an ear. If that isn't available, then I make sure David is settled in and draw a nice warm bath, light some candles, and listen to soothing music.

What is the best/worst piece of advice you have ever been given? Best piece of advice I received was from the neuropsychologist and that was to get all our affairs in order. Doing this has made it a lot easier to get things done like selling a vehicle in David's name and getting a home equity loan to do some moderate repairs to the home. It has been five years that he hasn't been inclined to attend to things around the house.

What is the best/worst thing you have learned about yourself? Best: Although I am a control-freak, I have learned patience and acceptance. It took me the better part of a year to get to the point that I "get it". I am able to separate the person from the disease. Worst: I am my worst critic. I am definitely too hard on myself. Need work on forgiving myself when I don't handle a situation in the best possible way, causing frustration, fear, or confusion to David.

What would you most like to tell someone who has become a caregiver? Accept that you will make mistakes, but as long as you are doing what you feel to be the best (given the situation/information) do not be hard on yourself.

What would you do if someone handed you $100,000? Save it, because I know that further along in the journey it will be needed for additional care.

What would you do with three extra hours a day? At this point of my journey, where my husband is still very much able to perform daily responsibilities, I do not have a lack of time.

What do you wish you had more of? Patience. Although I am better than a year ago, I still have my moments of frustration.

What are some easy things you do to relax or find joy? Read, puzzles, listen to music.

What is the best/worst question you have ever been asked? Best: "How are you holding up?" Most times the person asking this really gets it and is able to offer a much-needed ear to bend. Worst: "Is he doing better?" This definitely shows a lack of understanding exactly what this disease entails.

What are three things someone could do to help YOU (not your loved one, but you)? Minor repairs on the house (i.e. fix a leaking toilet, change a ceiling fan). Take my husband for an outing (i.e. lunch, fishing, car ride).

When was the last time you cried? I'm a crier. I pretty much cry every day, at least tear up every day.

Do you like yourself? I do. I know that I am not perfect, but I am confident that I am doing the best that I can for my husband at this phase of the journey. And although I do get down at time, I do not let myself stay there and I have ways of doing that.

What is the hardest thing you have faced? The lack of control over the situation. Early in the diagnosis I was able to handle it by making sure everything was in order, such as wills, power of attorney documents, and such. Now it just seems to be a waiting game – waiting for the next lost ability.

What is the one thing that no one can understand about your situation? Not all dementia is Alzheimer's. I have had to do a lot of education to family and friends because their first reaction was that he remembers so much. Once they viewed the videos and read the pamphlets, they then began to understand the complexity of FTD and were able to come up with examples of David exhibiting classic behaviors of the disease.

What is it that everyone should know, but no one wants to talk about? Everyone should know the impact this disease has on the entire family. And although the prognosis is dire, our loved ones still have aspects of their lives that are joyful (at least in the early-moderate stages). The stigma of dementia is causing a lot of relationships to end unnecessarily.

Do you have support from family? Friends? Church? Others? I do have some support from family and friends and faith community. Because of our relatively young age (57-58), many of my family and friends are still in the workforce, so have limited ability to provide physical support, but they do provide emotional and moral support.

What do you miss the most? Our dreams for retirement. His hugs. Our conversations.

Do you have a humorous story you would like to share? Although I do not have a story to tell, my son and I often times chuckle at the relationship between my grandson (5) and my husband. Many times, it is as though we are watching two 5-year-olds on a play date (even down to the minor arguments over the toys).

Anything else you would like to add? Education within the medical field about the various types of dementia is lacking. Although we were fortunate to find a neurologist experienced in FTD, there are many examples where lack of diagnosis has been detrimental to the families involved.

List any resources that you have found helpful in your journey. The AFTD website. The FTD support forum online. Facebook support groups: The FTD Spouse; Frontotemporal Dementia (FTD) Support Group Australia (and beyond); Dementia Care – Love, Laughter, Tears & Lessons with Gilly B; Caring of spouse with Dementia; Mother and Son's Journey with Dementia. Books: *What If It's Not Alzheimer's*; *The 36 Hour Day*. And all of Teepa Snow's videos.

DANA
Indians Rocks Beach, FL

"We will continue to survive."

Caree and age at diagnosis: Noel, 52
Diagnosis: bvFTD, July 16, 2015

Where do you find hope? Comfort? I find comfort and hope in church. I like to just sit and know that I am safe there, because I realize sometimes all I can do is pray. I find comfort and hope talking to my mom, sister, and my close friends. They don't judge, they listen. I find comfort being with my kids at night after he goes to bed. We go into "lockdown" and "lockout." At this time each night, we are free to be ourselves and not be criticized, micromanaged, belittled, or cussed at by the FTD person that used to be "Daddy Man."

What is one thing about caregiving (or you or others) that surprised you most? The one thing that has surprised me the most is the fact that I don't sweat the small stuff anymore, and I am, unfortunately, becoming hardened. I can go to work and be totally ON having had only four or five hours of sleep. I can fix things around the house. I can survive. I can be independent. I am not the perfectionist I once was either!

How do you take care of yourself? I take care of myself by praying. I have family and friends that let me just talk. I take walks. I laugh with my kids. I journal and keep track of everything going on with this disease. I pour myself into my kids and my teaching career. I promised myself a long time ago this monster (FTD) would never get me too.

What do you do when you hit bottom? When I hit rock bottom, I go to my laundry room and lock the door. Sometimes I call my mom or my sister. Sometimes I pray and scream and just talk to myself. I honestly try not to cry, because I am so scared if I start I won't be able to stop.

What is the best/worst piece of advice you have ever been given? I have had really good advice. Keep him away from money. Get a power of attorney. Take the keys away. Separate yourself from the disease. Remember this too shall pass, meaning that as hard as it is to believe, my life will not always be this way. Attitude is ninety-nine percent of almost everything, so don't give up. I don't recall any bad advice. Most people are just amazed at his behavior and decline and wonder how on earth the kids and I do this on a daily basis.

What is the best/worst thing you have learned about yourself? The best thing I have learned about myself is that I am an extremely strong woman. My kids love and support me. They swear they will never leave me alone to have to deal with this. We love each other and have the best bond. The worst thing I have learned about myself is I wonder if I put up with too much. At least I will never have to wonder if there was anything else I could have done. I can honestly say I have done all I know to do.

What would you most like to tell someone who has become a caregiver? I would tell that caregiver, "You are going to have good days and bad days, and it's not easy. Have a support system. Take care of your caree, but don't take what they say to heart, especially if it is bad, because every day is a new day for them and for you. Also, forget being a perfectionist. It's not happening with caregiving. Do your best. That's all you can do."

What would you do if someone handed you $100,000? With $100,000 I would pay off all my bills, take care of some needed "fixing" around the house, buy a new vehicle, and hire my elder care attorney with whom I consulted with last year, get Medicaid approved (doing this is a full-time job in itself, but I have been told I could qualify), and put my FTD spouse in the memory care facility where he desperately needs to be for his safety and well-being.

What would you do with three extra hours a day? I would sleep, spend more time with my kids and myself.

What do you wish you had more of? I wish I had more money and more time.

What are some easy things you do to relax or find joy?
1. I spend time with my kids.
2. I clean the house.
3. I talk to my friends and family.
4. I go to church and/or pray.
5. I read FB's the FTD Spouse's newsfeed.

These things get done, but the time spent with each depends on the day.

What is the best/worst question you have ever been asked? The number one question has always been, "How do you do this?" My answer has always been, "We all have our pile of $h!t! Some may choose to hide it, but we all have our own pile. I do it because I have to. I have not been given a choice." Is this the best question or the worst question? I don't know.

What are three things someone could do to help YOU (not your loved one, but you)? 1) To my family, come stay with me. Live here with me. Just be here. There are some days that I wish someone would just take over and let me sleep or go away. Respite is fine, but nothing gets done while I'm gone. I need help fixing things, paying bills, running errands, etc. 2) To friends and family, continue to pray for me all the time. 3) To my friends and family, keep listening to me!

When was the last time you cried? I honestly don't remember. I would love to though! I'm saving this for the end. I am so afraid if I start, I won't be able to stop.

Do you like yourself? I love myself! I am a strong person. I am very impressed with myself! My kids and family tell me I have it together.

What is the hardest thing you have faced? The hardest thing I have faced is watching my kids grow up with a father figure that they can only remember as being mean and insulting and uncaring. Another thing I have faced is listening to and watching the man I loved develop such a hatred toward me and our children for absolutely no other reason besides bvFTD. Then he wants to know why we are so impersonal and why the kids don't want to be around him….and then, I watch him and take care of him as he has seizures, declines, becomes confused, wanders off, goes into liver failure, hurts, and forgets.

What is the one thing that no one can understand about your situation? Yes, it is the disease talking! However, that does not take the hurt away! And, the big one…there is so much more to dementia than forgetfulness!

What is it that everyone should know, but no one wants to talk about? For the first years of this, before diagnosis, I hid the fact that I thought I was an abused wife because it was so embarrassing. I guess I thought it would just all go away and fix itself. I think when the diagnosis came we all felt empowered. It wasn't our fault anymore. Thank goodness he was rude and disoriented around his primary care physician. She got the diagnosis ball rolling.

Do you have support from family? Friends? Church? Others? I have support from all of the above, …. I am so, so blessed.

What do you miss the most? I miss my kids being able to talk to their Daddy. I miss them having a Daddy. They can't stand their father. Sadly, I can't blame them.

Do you have a humorous story you would like to share? This is an interesting question. I don't have any humorous stories to share. At the end of the day, when it's all said and done, I find no humor in this at all. Some days friends ask me how I am doing. Some days I smile and say I am fine, and other days I spill it. Some laugh at some of the stories I tell about what my FTD spouse has done. I understand they think it is funny. However, I don't think it is funny. I find no humor in this at all.

Anything else you would like to add? I am 52 years old. I am a veteran elementary school teacher. In 2010-11, my now FTD spouse started showing symptoms. My kids were just kids when this all started. The big things were MAJOR agitation, confusion, and unreasonable thinking. My son is now 20, and my daughter is now 13. My son attends college. He was an Eagle Scout at 14. He is a kitchen manager at a local restaurant. He is quite the artist, and he plays many different instruments. He earned his private pilot's license at the age of 19. He is a wonderful human being. My daughter is in middle school. She loves sports, art, and being with her friends. We are terribly scarred by this disease. We probably have PTSD. We've been told for years how pathetic we are as human beings by this FTD monster. We are surviving, and we will continue to survive. My son said it best to his little sister, "I sure wish you knew him the way he used to be."

List any resources that you have found helpful in your journey.

Family, friends, church, and the FTD Spouse Facebook page have all been lifesavers.

JIM
Barrington, IL

"Be ready to listen."

Caree and age at diagnosis: Joyce, 70
Diagnosis: Dementia, Winter 2012

Where do you find hope? Comfort? Through Christian friends and family.

What is one thing about caregiving (or you or others) that surprised you most? One of the things that surprised me was the number of people that are going through a similar situation to what I am going through once you start talking to them about it. Also, the amount of patience and understanding needed to be a caregiver and support the one I love.

How do you take care of yourself? In the beginning stages I would take my wife out with relatives who understood what the situation was and would spend time with Joyce while allowing me time to socialize with others and relax a bit. As the disease progressed, it became harder and harder to take Joyce out of the house. My children were concerned for my health and well-being as the disease progressed.

What do you do when you hit bottom? My children were a great support to me. They would help with meals and household things, allowing me the time I needed to take care of my wife. Before hitting bottom, you need to acknowledge that you can't do it alone and reach out to those you trust and love for help. If you wait too long, you limit your options.

What is the best/worst piece of advice you have ever been given? The best piece of advice I was given was that you have to learn to listen. Not just to the verbal communication, because that diminishes with dementia, but you have to watch for the non-verbal signs and you also have to realize how scared the person with the disease probably is, not understanding anything that is going on. Knowing that helps you to be more understanding and helped me to be more patient than I thought I could be.

What is the best/worst thing you have learned about yourself? I've learned that when you think you are doing your best, you need to think again, because you can probably be doing better. I have learned that I can't do it all myself and that I need to ask for help. The worst thing I learned about myself is that I don't like asking people for help.

What would you most like to tell someone who has become a caregiver? Be ready to listen. You are not number one in your life, but you do need to take care of yourself in order to take care of someone else. You are not number one, but you are not last either.

What would you do if someone handed you $100,000? I am not sure what I would do with $100,000. I would not spend it. I would invest some and donate some to a worthy cause that helps others.

What would you do with three extra hours a day? Take a nap.

What do you wish you had more of? Time with my wife before she had dementia.

What are some easy things you do to relax or find joy? Take a nap, listen to music, spend time with people I love, watch John Wayne movies (or other Westerns) and go to church.

What is the best/worst question you have ever been asked? No question is a bad question when someone is sincere in asking it.

What are three things someone could do to help YOU (not your loved one, but you)? Mow my grass, listen to me, and spend time with me.

When was the last time you cried? The last time I thought about the woman that I love.

Do you like yourself? Most of the time.

What is the hardest thing you have faced? My wife developing dementia.

What is the one thing that no one can understand about your situation? How much I love my wife even though she looks at me like I am a stranger to her.

What is it that everyone should know, but no one wants to talk about? You should always tell the people you love that you love them, even when you are angry with them. You never know what the future holds.

Do you have support from family? Friends? Church? Others? Yes, my kids have been a great support. My extended family has been encouraging. Friends and members of my church have been there to pray for, offer advice from their experiences with the disease, and spend time with us.

What do you miss the most? Having my wife and best friend with me every day to discuss life with.

Do you have a humorous story you would like to share? Your hearing is as good as you want it to be. One day my wife was on the tractor and I was in the bucket painting the garage. The kids leaned in to ask her quietly if they should stop and get custard. Over the tractor motor and my work, I responded YES!!!

List any resources that you have found helpful in your journey.

The best resource I have found is talking to people who have had loved ones of their own go through this process. All cases are different, but human nature is the same and we can learn how to better handle things from people who have been through it and share with us how they handled it. It also gives you an idea of what may be coming so you can best prepare yourself.

KIRSTIN
New Hartford, NY

"You are enough."

Caree and age at diagnosis: Mike, 42
Diagnosis: PPA/FTD, September 2017

Where do you find hope? Comfort? I find hope in those glimmers of who my husband once was. When he watches baseball, or responds to a joke, or sometimes even fires one of his famous zingers, it's almost like he's still here. I find comfort in the fact that, most days, he doesn't seem to know what's happening to him. He's relatively calm, easy going, and happy. I'm lucky he doesn't lash out or become depressed.

What is one thing about caregiving (or you or others) that surprised you most? One thing that surprised me, I think, was that people don't really understand. Unless they spend time with our family, they think he is fine. Then something happens where a friend or family member is around us for a longer period of time and I hear, "I had no idea it was this bad." And in that, I think, there's loneliness. No one really knows your situation because they don't live it day in and day out like you do.

How do you take care of yourself? Before my husband's stroke (April 2013, four and a half years before FTD diagnosis), I had lost about 60 pounds and was working on being the healthiest I could be. With the stress of these past five years, it all came back. So, I'm working on eating healthy again, and I recently went to a rowing class that was challenging, but fun. Other ways I take care of myself are seeing a therapist, belonging to two caregiver support groups on Facebook, and making sure I get to see my girlfriends around once a month. Oh, and at my last doctor's appointment, I asked for medication to help with the overwhelming nature of my life (recently at work, I cried because I didn't have a spoon for my lunch!).

What do you do when you hit bottom? I have a best friend I can call at any time, who's also my cousin. She's great for venting. Some days I lay in bed and pull the covers over my head for a few hours. But with three kids and my husband to care for, I really don't have the time to wallow. I try to stay positive most of the time, and to find the humor in everyday life.

What is the best/worst piece of advice you have ever been given? The best piece of advice I've ever been given is that I have the right to grieve. I spent the year or two after the stroke struggling with the feeling that I should be grateful that I still had my husband, and my kids still had their father (they were 9, 6, and 3 at the time). My life was thrown a complete curve ball, and I was trying to be grateful. My friend pointed out that we had all lost something, and that it was okay to grieve. Once I began the grieving process, my mindset started to shift. I'll always love my husband, and I'll always take care of him, but the man I married is no longer here. I miss him. Going through the grieving process also helped me when he started to decline, because I was able to be slightly more objective about his needs and the needs of the rest of the family.

The worst piece of advice was probably the armchair physician type of advice - the people that suddenly seem to know exactly what they're talking about, or who profess to know more than the doctors.

What is the best/worst thing you have learned about yourself? I'm pretty strong. I'm capable of running a household and taking care of 'man' chores (dispensing with mice is the worst thing I've had to face) and running the household budget. My patience is fairly strong; I feel like I'm usually even-keeled and kind.

The worst thing is that when I do lose my patience, I'm really not nice and my mouth suddenly starts spewing things that normally don't come out of it. In those moments I know I need a few minutes to myself to come back down, take some deep breaths, and refocus.

What would you most like to tell someone who has become a caregiver? First of all, I'm sorry you have to do this. It's hard. It's thankless and it's lonely. But it also is who you are. Only good people take on this task of caregiving. You also need to make sure that you give care to yourself as well as your loved one. It doesn't do anyone any good for you to allow yourself to get run down. Reach out for support; it's out there. You are not alone.

What would you do if someone handed you $100,000? Pay off my van and my mortgage, take my family to Disney World, and then go right back to work and our life as we know it. Work for me is my respite care.

What would you do with three extra hours a day? I'd like to say I'd be productive and work on getting my house organized, but I'd probably just relax with my phone, a book, or Netflix.

What do you wish you had more of? Time with my husband before the changes, and money.

What are some easy things you do to relax or find joy? Spend time outside in the spring, go to the beach, hang out with my kids, go out with my girlfriends, be with my parents.

What is the best/worst question you have ever been asked? Best: How can I help you today? Worst: Why don't you just let his mother take care of him?

What are three things someone could do to help YOU (not your loved one, but you)? Take him out during the day while I'm at work (I wouldn't worry as much), schedule a coffee date with me, offer to take my kids after school once in a while.

When was the last time you cried? Hah, Yesterday? No, probably last week.

What is the hardest thing you have faced? Bankruptcy paperwork, disability paperwork, Medicaid paperwork.

What is the one thing that no one can understand about your situation? I'm no stronger than anyone else. I just do what I have to do.

What is it that everyone should know, but no one wants to talk about? This is hard. And it's unfair.

Do you have support from family? Friends? Church? Others? My parents, my in-laws (now just my mother-in-law), and friends and colleagues.

What do you miss the most? My husband was so smart and funny. I miss having a partner. I miss being able to share the raising of our kids and the highs and lows of life. I miss physical touch.

Do you have a humorous story you would like to share? I've found things in the most interesting places: a sandwich with one bite out of it in the freezer, a ceramic bowl in the toilet, candy wrappers stuffed into the paper towel tube. Sometimes life is like a secret scavenger hunt in my house. We never know what we're going to find or where we'll find it.

Anything else you would like to add? For young caregivers with kids, find time for them to be with you and express how they're feeling. Acknowledge their experiences in this situation. Also, make sure you take care of you. It's okay for you to do for yourself or to let your house be a little messy. Taking care of everyone is enough. You are enough.

List any resources that you have found helpful in your journey. I found some community agencies that helped me with paperwork and are currently working with me to get my husband into day care while I'm at work.

MAJA
Moncks Corner, SC

"Have those big girl panties ready!"

Caree and age at diagnosis: Russ, 50
Diagnosis: FTD, February 2015

Where do you find hope? Comfort? My faith, friends, family; the fact that I am still young (relatively speaking – 48, he is 52).

What is one thing about caregiving (or you or others) that surprised you most? I knew it was hard…just being powerless as the disease progresses.

How do you take care of yourself? Not very well really. I have had to become very selfish which is very hard for me. I have had to learn to do what I want to do when possible with or without husband. I do sew as a hobby when I can. I like to walk when I can with a friend.

What do you do when you hit bottom? Cry. Pray. Take a break from the house, him, and child in college (who is bipolar manic and severely ADHD). Take Ativan. Glass of wine doesn't hurt either.

What is the best/worst piece of advice you have ever been given? Worst - Try this remedy or that. Hopefully it will improve. I just reply it is past remedies and it is terminal. I have had to get downright nasty and in someone's face (as politely as a Southern woman can) and tell them no essential oils, no vitamins, whatever, etc. several times.

What is the best/worst thing you have learned about yourself? I have had so many people tell me that I am a good person to have put up with everything I have, that not many would do that. I am uncomfortable with people telling me that, but understand as I have had to become very selfish, so I am not consumed by the needed care, apathy, lack of empathy, etc. I have amazing friends. I try to rely on my faith more and more. Ativan can be my friend!

What would you most like to tell someone who has become a caregiver? Have those big girl panties ready! You cannot do this alone. Get POA's or whatever asap. Find support groups online. The ones I belong to have been instrumental in keeping me sane and not feeling alone.

What would you do if someone handed you $100,000? Fix my house so husband is safer, get a small camper so we can travel a little while he still half-way knows what is going on. Pay bills with the rest.

What would you do with three extra hours a day? While someone cleans my house during those hours, I would sew, relax, have peace without having to listen for the next thing to happen. Totally different than having to keep an ear out for young children. Can't really explain, but it is different.

What do you wish you had more of? Time and money so we can do some of what we planned to do when we retired. Hard to know you won't be able to celebrate certain milestone wedding anniversaries, see future grandchildren grow up, etc.

What are some easy things you do to relax or find joy? Get with friends, sew, read, watch TV series, get outside/garden.

What is the best/worst question you have ever been asked? Best – "What can I do to help?" And they actually do help. Worst – "Why are you still with him?"

What are three things someone could do to help YOU (not your loved one, but you)? Back massage – deep tissue – seriously! Clean my house regularly. Be there to go to a movie, lunch, etc.

When was the last time you cried? Last night. At least every couple of days.

Do you like yourself? Yes, but feel guilty for wanting an intimate relationship again, guilty about being selfish to save my sanity. Guilty of having to do or not allowing certain things so that I and the children will have a future.

What is the hardest thing you have faced? Watching this strong, independent, compassionate man disappear before my eyes daily and having to help the children deal with it too. Also, having to know and be ready to restrict activities.

What is the one thing that no one can understand about your situation? They don't see the subtle changes since they don't live with him. The nuances are hard to see. And that there is no cure.

What is it that everyone should know, but no one wants to talk about? That he can't do what he used to and doesn't believe it or understand why…loss of intimacy, but he can hold a perfectly normal conversation to a certain point so that everyone else thinks you are making it all up.

Do you have support from family? Friends? Church? Others? I feel that I have been extremely supported. Now, his family, I don't think are totally convinced. A brother and a sister have been here once, but he was still in very early stages. The brother thinks that Russ can move up there with him and he and his wife can take care of him (like they did their mother when she had cancer), so I don't eventually place him in a veteran's home. Hell, no.

What do you miss the most? My best friend.

Anything else you would like to add? That I feel guilty for trying to make plans for the future since I still have five years until retirement and must work full time. Although I do work from home as an online teacher, he gets very jealous of the fact that I am on the computer. I am scared that I won't find someone to be with. I almost wish that there was a way for him to be able to end things on his terms when he wants to, since he has expressed that he doesn't want to become that helpless person and doesn't want the kids to see him like that.

List any resources that you have found helpful in your journey. Online support groups. Lawyers and eldercare attorney. Outstanding friends.

MAUREEN
Seaford, DE

"I try to only live today."

Caree and age at diagnosis: Tom, 58
Diagnosis: bvFTD, May 2012

Where do you find hope? Comfort? I find hope in my faith. There is no hope that a miracle will happen, but there is hope that I will make it through this horrible journey. I also find comfort in the support groups that I am a part of on Facebook.

What is one thing about caregiving (or you or others) that surprised you most? The thing that surprised me the most is my strength. My ability to get up every day and take care of my husband, change his diapers. I have also learned that things I thought were important to me before my husband's diagnosis do not mean anything to me today. There are times I fall apart, but I go to bed every night and pray for strength to make it through the next day.

How do you take care of yourself? I have hired someone to come in and be with my husband on Thursdays. It is my 'sanity day'. I try to do whatever I think I need on that day. Sometimes I get a pedicure, sometimes I sit by the river with a coffee and a book, and sometimes I go shopping. I always come home refreshed, although the time goes by quickly.

What do you do when you hit bottom? I cry, I have a drink, I sit in the hot tub and talk to the moon and God. I ask Him to help me get through this. Sometimes, I even get mad at Him because of my situation, but then I realize that I could not get through this without His help. I also go to my support groups on-line and read what other caregivers are going through. There are highs and lows, tears and laughter displayed in their posts and it always makes me certain that I am not alone. I also keep a gratitude journal. I try to start every day with three things that I am grateful for because I truly believe that there is always something that makes me grateful.

What is the best/worst piece of advice you have ever been given? The worst advice is when my husband was first diagnosed, I was told to find a facility for him. In my heart, I never want to put my husband in a facility because I believe in treating others as you want to be treated. I never, NEVER want to live in a nursing home facility. I am not saying I will never have to place Tom, I am saying I don't want to. I think I will know when I can longer do what I am doing, and I will take the appropriate steps. The best advice is to not overthink FTD and what could or could not happen. Take each day or even one hour as it comes. I try to only live today. Things that I would worry about could or could not happen. So, I try to just focus on the current situation.

What is the best/worst thing you have learned about yourself? The best thing is that I am strong and empathetic. The worst thing is that I am not as empathetic as I could be, and I don't want to be strong anymore. As my husband continues to decline, I dream of an easier way of life. Not having to take Depends and changes of clothes with me everywhere. I dream of not having to make all the decisions. I dream of my old life.

What would you most like to tell someone who has become a caregiver? I am so sorry that you have to go through this journey that is sometimes hell. I pray that you can survive this horrible disease. Please try to find a support group and be good to yourself. By that I do not just mean doing things that rejuvenate you but forgive yourself. You are doing the very best at this sometimes impossible job.

What would you do if someone handed you $100,000? I would try to find someone who is an FTD spouse caregiver and help them in some way. I would also invest the money so that when or if the time comes that I need to put Tom in a nursing home, I would not have the financial worries that I have now.

What would you do with three extra hours a day? I really have no clue. I dream of having extra time, but the truth is I have forgotten who I am and what makes me happy. All the dreams I had of retirement are gone. If, God willing, I survive this horrible, evil disease, I will have to take time to find out who I am and what will make me happy.

What do you wish you had more of? Naturally, I wish I had more financial freedom. I would be able to pay for additional hours that I could have more sanity time for me.

What are some easy things you do to relax or find joy? 1) I play games on the computer; my favorite is pixel art and coloring. It relaxes me. 2) I sit in the hot tub with a Bloody Mary and look at the moon and the stars. I look at the planes and dream of going somewhere relaxing and fun. 3) I go outside and walk, and then get a cup of coffee or tea. I take Tom with me now, but he walks at a snail's pace, but it is good to get out on nice days. 4) I go on the internet and go to Amazon, Wayfair, Overstock.com, etc. and I start to put things in my shopping cart, price is no object.... I buy whatever fits my mood of the day.

Then I go to the shopping cart and delete everything. It is good to dream. 5) Every day we go driving, as Tom was a driver's ed teacher and he loves riding. He no longer talks but we put on his hymns and he sings. It is good to hear his voice.

What is the best/worst question you have ever been asked? Best, "Is there anything I can do for you?" Worst, "Is your husband getting better?"

What are three things someone could do to help YOU (not your loved one, but you)? 1) Paint some walls and do some maintenance work around the house. 2) Bring me dinner; I am so tired of doing all the cooking. 3) Watch Tom for a while so I can just take a nap.

When was the last time you cried? I get teary every day. I am not really a crier. I don't usually cry if I am upset or angry. I cry when people are kind and thoughtful.

Do you like yourself? Most days I like myself. There are many times I am disappointed in myself, especially when Tom gets on my nerves and I am short with him. But most days, I think I am doing the very best job I possibly can.

What is the hardest thing you have faced? Loss. When I was 20, my father who had just turned 50 died of a massive heart attack. My husband at the age of 58 was diagnosed with bvFTD and little by little I am losing him. Both losses are heartbreaking.

What is the one thing that no one can understand about your situation? How lonely this journey is. I have lost my husband and best friend. I have lost our group of friends because it is becoming impossible to take Tom out in a group. I quit my job so I could be full-time caregiver to Tom. I know it was the best thing to do, but I lost that identity. FTD is just a series of losses, the worst loss being our hopes and dreams.

What is it that everyone should know, but no one wants to talk about? How horrible it is to take care of someone who no longer knows how to pee, poop, or clean themselves.

Do you have support from family? Friends? Church? Others? I have tremendous support of my family. We are the fourth generation to build on the family farm. My son and his wife built right next door. You can drive one mile down my road and see no one but family. What I thought 20 years ago was a curse has turned into a blessing.

What do you miss the most? Intimacy, talking, friendship, just enjoying being together. I started dating my husband when I was 16 and was married at the age of 20. I never dreamed this is how we would end up.

ANITA
North Royalton, OH

"We are all forever changed."

Caree and age at diagnosis: Richard, 68
Diagnosis: bvFTD/PPA, July 2015

Where do you find hope? Comfort? There is no hope until there is a treatment or cure. Until then the FTD path is of cruel brain atrophy which ends in death before it robs victims of who they are. It challenges caregivers past limits they never dreamed or imagined. We are all forever changed.

I found a Facebook closed group called FTD Spouses where there are others like myself. They understand like no one else in my small circle of family support. This group provides the ability to say what we are truly feeling without judgment. No matter what I have written, there are others who have been through the same or similar. They are my lifeline of sanity.

My strength comes from my faith in God.

What is one thing about caregiving (or you or others) that surprised you most? I never imagined the loneliness I would experience as a caregiver to my husband. This is a quote I saved because it says it all, "A diagnosis of cancer and everyone rushes to help…Dementia and everyone disappears."

How do you take care of yourself? I see a therapist, a psychiatrist, and take medication to help with my depression and anxiety. I do a poor job of physically caring for myself. I don't follow-through with making medical or dentist appointments, I eat poorly, sleep is difficult, and I have little motivation.

What do you do when you hit bottom? I cry uncontrollably and feel my life is completely hopeless. It doesn't matter if I am alive or not. I withdraw from everyone and everything. It is difficult to get out of bed and sleep is my escape.

What is the best/worst piece of advice you have ever been given? Best advice: Better to be proactive than reactive. I researched and read everything I could on FTD. This enabled me to be aware of the changes/stages of FTD. Where that played the greatest role was visiting memory care before placement was necessary. I understood there were waiting lists so I wanted to have my husband on that list so placement would be when I was ready, not waiting for the facility's availability.

Worst advice: After FTD diagnosis, my husband had a prostate biopsy which indicated he had a slow, progressive cancer. The urologist wanted my husband to follow up with a prostate scan and continue with prostate biopsies to monitor the cancer's progression. My husband's primary care doctor and I agreed that the prep and procedures would be too difficult with my husband's dementia. We also agreed treating and monitoring the cancer would be to lengthen his life living with a degenerative brain disease. That would not enhance his quality of life.

What is the best/worst thing you have learned about yourself? Best: To my disbelief, how strong a person I am. Worst: The behaviors and compulsions from FTD brought out the worst in me as a person and wife. I easily angered and felt his actions and lack of empathy were deliberate. This went against the person I am.

What would you most like to tell someone who has become a caregiver? To run away as fast as you can and never look back (kidding). I would tell them to research and educate themselves. Educate their families and friends as they will need a great deal of support from them. To find an elder care attorney to get their legal and financial affairs in order as soon as possible. With their neurologist's guidance, take away driving privileges. Join caregiver support group meetings. Lastly, be proactive and not reactive.

What would you do if someone handed you $100,000? Travel to my husband's bucket list destinations before the dementia worsens. Find the absolute best memory care facility without the financial aspect forcing the choice.

What would you do with three extra hours a day? I would take time for myself. Meet friends for lunch, go shopping, go to the movies, a museum, anything that will distract me.

What do you wish you had more of? I wish I had more time with my husband before FTD struck him, struck me, struck us.

What are some easy things you do to relax or find joy? This is a tough question for me to answer. The first year after diagnosis I spent crying. I was incapable of any joy or relaxation. 1. Spend time with my 1-year-old granddaughter – the greatest joy I have. 2. I enjoy my quiet time and find I prefer to be by myself now that my husband is in a memory care facility. 3. Watching TV or movies. 4. Reading books.

What is the best/worst question you have ever been asked? Best question: A new woman attending a caregivers' support group wanted to talk to me (in her words) "How do you do it? You have it all together." My immediate thought was, "You have to be kidding me?" Apparently, my outward appearance and composure makes it appear I have it under control. Inside I'm a mess. Worst question: After my husband went into the memory care facility, a male neighbor asked me, "When is your husband coming home?" Really? As if I don't feel bad enough as it is that he needed placement, and I was the one who placed him. I was taken aback and weakly explained why he wasn't coming home. The look on my neighbor's face I interpreted as I was an awful person that I didn't keep him home. Guilt set in.

What are three things someone could do to help YOU (not your loved one, but you)?
1. To call me on a regular basis to check in on me.
2. Invite me somewhere, be it lunch, dinner, movie, etc.
3. It would warm my heart if my husband had visitors at the memory care facility other than myself. It saddens me that the people who know him have forgotten him.

When was the last time you cried? Today.

Do you like yourself? Yes, I do, but, as I previously stated, living with my husband's bvFTD made me angry and often impatient with him. By nature, I have great empathy and understanding. That went out the window with his FTD.

What is the hardest thing you have faced? The placement of my husband in a memory care facility. I cannot begin to describe the guilt, grief, and sadness. I will say no wife should ever have to do that to their husband. This is a whole different level than placing a parent or grandparent.

What is the one thing that no one can understand about your situation? The depth of pain that comes from watching your once vibrant and active husband lose everything that made him who he is. His behavior now is of a small child. This first time I watched him at the facility hold hands with a caretaker to walk and guide him down the hall, it broke my already broken heart.

What is it that everyone should know, but no one wants to talk about? I wish my family and friends took the time to read up on FTD. To simply know what it is and what it is capable of doing to a person. And for the love of God, it is NOT Alzheimer's!

Do you have support from family? Friends? Church? Others? I have varying levels of support from family and friends. Prior to my husband's placement, his sister who lives out of state called or texted me every day or so. She was my greatest support. Now that he resides in a facility, I rarely hear from her. I guess all my problems have been solved. (I am being facetious.) At this time my greatest support comes from the Facebook group of FTD Spouses. They are my lifeline of sanity.

What do you miss the most? To identify what I miss the most, I cannot. There is far too much to write. What I can say is I miss the person who was my lover, my companion, and my best friend for thirty years.

Do you have a humorous story you would like to share? There is not a lot of humor as a caregiver to a husband with bvFTD, but now that he is placed, there have been a few. My husband has become that person who goes into other residents' rooms and takes things. He gathers blankets and brings them to his room. This past week I walked in his room to find a huge mound of blankets at his feet, as tall as the side of his bed. He had removed every sheet, blanket, and bedspread from his roommate's bed and added it to his blanket pile.

DEBBIE
Hornell, NY

"You can't do this alone."

Caree and age at diagnosis: Casey, 56
Diagnosis: bvFTD, March 2015

Where do you find hope? Comfort? I find hope and comfort in my true friends and family who have stood by me throughout our journey with bvFTD.

What is one thing about caregiving (or you or others) that surprised you most? How difficult caregiving really is! I am an RN but had never been a full-time caregiver. When my husband was starting to get worse, I had a full-time job, and also took care of him full-time. Hardest job I have ever done. Looking back, I am amazed that I was able to do both and function.

How do you take care of yourself? When I was caregiving, my retreat was my hot tub. It was my thinking spot, relaxing spot, crying spot, and all-around haven from caregiving stress.

What do you do when you hit bottom? Talk with others who understand. The FTD Spouse website was truly the answer to my prayers. It was through talking with others who were/are going through the same thing that I am/was that I was able to work it through, realize that I am not alone, and find love and understanding on this most difficult of journeys.

What is the best/worst piece of advice you have ever been given? When it came time to place my husband there was a lot of guilt, even though I had done my best and had no choice in the matter. I was given great advice by other spouses, such as that I was not doing it to him, but for him, and that it was not my decision, but disease progress that made placement necessary. That really helped me to understand that the decision to place was really made for me, and out of my control.

What is the best/worst thing you have learned about yourself? That I am much stronger than I ever thought I was. That I am able to love with all of my heart and soul and continue to do this despite circumstances that would likely extinguish the love from other relationships. That I am capable of much more than I ever believed possible.

What would you most like to tell someone who has become a caregiver? Get support, whether it be from family, friends, or a wonderful support group that you can relate to. Be ready for some family/friends to step away, but others to step up. You will learn who your true supporters really are during this time. You can't do this alone!

What would you do if someone handed you $100,000? Probably retire earlier than planned. Since my caregiving experience is now over, what I have learned most is that life is indeed short. You need to live now, because the future is not guaranteed. I'd also give some to my children, to help make their life journeys a little bit easier.

What would you do with three extra hours a day? When I was caregiving, three extra hours a day would have been wonderful. I probably would have spent more time getting respite for myself, as caregiver stress can be huge. If possible, I probably would have used it to sleep, as that can be in short supply when you are caregiving for someone with dementia.

What do you wish you had more of? When I was caregiving and working full-time nights, I wish I could have taken a leave of absence from my job in order to just take care of my husband. Time was at such a premium, and I always felt like it was a monumental balancing act to continue doing both. Looking back, I truly don't know how I did it.

What are some easy things you do to relax or find joy? Some things that I did that helped were to talk with, commiserate, and problem-solve with other FTD spouses, spend time with family, relax in my hot tub every night for 15-30 minutes, get respite when I could, and journal.

What is the best/worst question you have ever been asked? It used to really bother me when people would say things like, "How do you ever do it?" or "I could never do it." Truth is, I didn't have a choice. Who would choose to have their spouse get dementia? Worst question/comment ever.

What are three things someone could do to help YOU (not your loved one, but you)? 1. Offer to take my LO somewhere. Anywhere. He would love it, and so would I. 2. Bring dinner one night. 3. Be a good friend. Don't be afraid to keep being a friend. Don't run away just because my spouse has dementia. (This goes for LO's friends as well.) On this note, see #1.

When was the last time you cried? Since dementia entered my life, I've cried at least daily. Sometimes way more than daily. It is a very sad disease, where we grieve constantly. My husband just died a few weeks ago, so of course, I am still crying. I cry in my car, in my hot tub, and sometimes when I really don't want to, such as when I am with other people. I try to keep my crying private.

Do you like yourself? Most of the time. I didn't at times when I lost my patience with my husband. I think, overall, I did a pretty good job of taking care of him, though, and am proud to say that I did the best I could, and loved him well until the end, despite all of the behaviors, upheaval, and difficulty that bvFTD threw at me.

What is the hardest thing you have faced? The behaviors and difficulty of dealing with the disease was extremely hard, but I have to say that the hardest thing was, of course, the death of my husband. The dying process itself was emotionally excruciating to go through. Being alone and knowing that I will never again see him on this earth is very difficult for me to deal with right now.

What is the one thing that no one can understand about your situation? If you haven't gone through it, you have no idea how hard it really all is. Trying to work and go on with life as if nothing is wrong, when everything is wrong. Putting on a game face and dying inside. I have done this since he was diagnosed in 2015. It is exhausting.

What is it that everyone should know, but no one wants to talk about? How hard this all really is on a caregiver. How caregivers really need support, but more often than not, don't get it.

Do you have support from family? Friends? Church? Others? My family has been wonderful. My husband had some friends that stuck by him/us, but others that fell away. I am immensely grateful for those friends and family who stayed. They were angels on earth. I will never forget their loyalty to us.

What do you miss the most? I miss our life before bvFTD. I miss talking to and being with my husband. I miss holding him and cuddling with him. I miss having someone to come home to and share my day with. I so miss being a couple. I miss "us".

Do you have a humorous story you would like to share? A story that I was thinking of today that made me laugh: Casey said to me one morning, "I think I ate some cat treats last night. And you know what, they weren't half bad." Only with dementia! We both got a good laugh out of that one.

List any resources that you have found helpful in your journey.
The FTD Spouse website was invaluable to me. When I had to apply for Medicaid (when Casey went into the nursing home), the Office for the Aging was very helpful. A few books that were helpful

during this journey for me were *Ambiguous Loss* and *What If It Isn't Alzheimer's?*

LAURA
Carlisle, MA

"Do not be a martyr."

Caree and age at diagnosis: Michael, 63
Diagnosis: bvFTD, 2014

Where do you find hope? Comfort? My comfort comes from the support we have had from loving family and friends. Our network has rallied to help us with love and support. My hope is that my husband continues to have no idea of the havoc this disease has had on him. He was a proud man who can no longer do the simplest of tasks. He has no idea his life is so different; that gives me hope that the power of this disease has not had the power to destroy his idea of who he is.

What is one thing about caregiving (or you or others) that surprised you most? I never considered myself a caregiver.... I am so surprised that I can do what I do, such as cleaning him up after being incontinent. I am surprised that I am so patient with him. I am also surprised at how protective I am of his dignity and my intolerance of other people's negative reaction to his bizarre behavior.

How do you take care of yourself? I work; I pay for help; I see my friends. We have been fortunate to be able to afford for the care of my husband, though it has financially hurt us. He is now being cared for at the VA hospital and life is easier for me now. Though I miss him terribly, I am sleeping at night and no longer using our retirement money for his daily care.

What do you do when you hit bottom? I remind myself that this disease was a small price to pay for the wonderful marriage I had. My husband was a fabulous husband and father and my best friend for over 35 years. I still consider myself the lucky one!

What is the best/worst piece of advice you have ever been given? Stay in the moment was the best advice. The worst advice was going to a support group meeting; it scared the heck out of me.

What is the best/worst thing you have learned about yourself? The best thing I learned was that gratitude is a great way of looking at things; the worst thing I learned about myself is that I eat when I am stressed and can't control binge eating when I am nervous. I have gained 20 pounds since my husband's diagnosis.

What would you most like to tell someone who has become a caregiver? Everyone says take care of yourself. When people told me that, I thought, "How the hell am I supposed to do that?" I have learned you need to ask for help so, when someone says, "What can I do for you?" reply, "Can you sit with my loved one? Can you shop for me? Can you pick something up for me? Can you have lunch with me?" People really want to help, do not be a martyr; give people direction on ways they can help.

What would you do if someone handed you $100,000? I would donate a portion to FTD research because no family should have to go through this horrible disease. I would re-fund my retirement accounts.

What would you do with three extra hours a day? Sleep!

What do you wish you had more of? Time. This disease has shown me how fast time goes by. I blinked, and my husband got sick; 38 years flew by. I wish I had more conversation with my husband when he had his full mind. I have so much I need to say to him, so many things I need to consult with him about; I always thought we would have time to wrap our lives up, to say what would you want…if…I need to know how to live without him from his perspective.

What are some easy things you do to relax or find joy? Eat, work, spend time with friends, spend time with family, tell my husband how wonderful he is and how much I love him.

What is the best/worst question you have ever been asked? "Will you get remarried?" was the worst question; I am still married (sort of). The best question was, "What would Dad want for you?"

What are three things someone could do to help YOU (not your loved one, but you)? Someone to visit without me paying them; volunteers to help with my yard and with the snow; gift certificates to get my nails done; a massage, hairdresser, and little luxuries for me.

When was the last time you cried? Today.

Do you like yourself? Yes, I like myself a lot.

What is the hardest thing you have faced? Living without my partner; not completing our plans together.

What is the one thing that no one can understand about your situation? The loneliness.

What is it that everyone should know, but no one wants to talk about? Timeline. How long to death? What does death look like?

What do you miss the most? Conversation, companionship.

Anything else you would like to add? FTD SUCKS!

List any resources that you have found helpful in your journey. Facebook support groups, a wonderful neurologist, and his staff.

LINDA
Tempe, AZ

"I miss my companion."

Caree and age at diagnosis: Randy, 60
Diagnosis: bvFTD, April 2014

Where do you find hope? Comfort? My relationship with Jesus Christ…my dependency on Him. Psalm 18 ~ "The Lord is my rock, my fortress and my deliverer, my God is my rock, in whom I take refuge, my shield and the horn of my salvation, my stronghold."

What is one thing about caregiving (or you or others) that surprised you most? When close friends and family disappeared. Feeling so isolated and alone.

How do you take care of yourself? By working 30 hours a week while my husband is at an adult day care. I feel removed from my personal life while I work. I also attend a women's Bible study that nourishes my hurting heart with the truth of God's Word.

What do you do when you hit bottom? I cry out to God for help and healing. I read the Psalms. I call a friend and we pray together.

What is the best/worst piece of advice you have ever been given? "If you've seen one person with FTD, you've seen one." (Geri Hall) Also, hire an elder-law attorney.

What is the best/worst thing you have learned about yourself? That I have patience, that nothing bothered me after my husband was diagnosed; and that while I thought I was not caregiver material, I actually am, but only because of God's help. The worst thing I learned about myself…not trusting God, and that knowing I have no control over this disease nor my kids lack of contact; I have an overwhelming desire to control everything else…desperate to have everything else predictable, routine, and normal.

What would you most like to tell someone who has become a caregiver? Accept, be patient and kind. Pray for God's strength and love to flow through you. Surround yourself with trusted truth-tellers that encourage you, inspire you, remind you of your identity in Christ. Process your journey with a qualified counselor. Ask for help. Memorize Scriptures that you can repeat over and over in the middle of the night when you wake up anxious, fearful, and lonely.

What would you do if someone handed you $100,000? FTD research, reserve the best facility for future placement, donate to ministries, buy a brand-new vehicle, vacation in the Canadian Rockies, Lake Louise, Banff.

What would you do with three extra hours a day? Hiking, lunch with a friend, sessions with a qualified counselor.

What do you wish you had more of? Time with friends. Trips to visit family in another state. Peace, joy and contentment, trusting God more and more through all the changes.

What are some easy things you do to relax or find joy? Listen to music, Netflix, study God's Word, walking, embroidery/sewing projects with a friend.

What is the best/worst question you have ever been asked? Best question? "How are you doing Linda? How can I come along side you in this unexpected journey?" Worst question? Ignorant about this type of dementia, assuming the onset is memory – asking if he still knows who I am.

What are three things someone could do to help YOU (not your loved one, but you)? 1. Letting me know they are thinking of me, praying for me…either through a text, voicemail, email, or an actual call. 2. Offer to bring a meal or help with a home maintenance project. 3. Take me on a long, much-needed road trip to get out of the city for the day.

When was the last time you cried? This morning after a major diarrhea clean up. Exhausting, heartbreaking.

Do you like yourself? Yes, I do…but then at times I don't…when I am weary and tired and feeling like I should be doing more for my husband.

What is the hardest thing you have faced? The reality that I am facing the future alone.

What is the one thing that no one can understand about your situation? Watching the love of your life slowly dying.

What is it that everyone should know, but no one wants to talk about? That caregivers need help, balance and time with family and friends. Yes, our loved one has a terminal disease, but we are ok. We have needs, hopes and dreams…and no one to share them with.

Do you have support from family? Friends? Church? Others? I have support from my church and a small group of friends and my sisters. My children who are 35, 33, and 28 are not a support.

What do you miss the most? My love language is acts of service, so I miss my companion, helpmate, doing projects together, fixing stuff. I miss the road trips, sharing our hopes and dreams and adding to our bucket list of adventures as we grow old together.

Do you have a humorous story you would like to share? I recently bought some all-natural dog treats, other than the usual hard dog biscuits. Dumped the entire bag in the jar on the counter. My husband got up during the night and ate the whole bag. Thankfully, chicken and carrots and sweet potato dog treats. But still…

RITA
Livingston, WI

"The uncertainty is one of the hardest things about this disease."

Caree and age at diagnosis: Chuck, 62
Diagnosis: bvFTD, June 2016

What is one thing about caregiving (or you or others) that surprised you most? The thing that surprises me most about being a caregiver is simply how hard it is. There are so many factors that others aren't aware of, such as, you are the only one who can take care of anything; the shopping, bills, appointments, cleaning, cooking, laundry, yard work, repairs…the list is endless.

How do you take care of yourself? I make it a point to maintain friendships and get out of the house occasionally without my spouse. Non-caregivers don't realize how important it is for caregivers to get a break; how important it is to maintain those friendships.

What do you do when you hit bottom? When I hit bottom, I have a good cry and get it out of my system. Then I make myself remember the man he used to be and how much I loved him; how he deserves to have the person he loves and counts on to be there for him in his scary, unfamiliar world. That puts things back into perspective for me.

What is the best/worst piece of advice you have ever been given? I don't know if it's advice or not, but the worst thing someone can say to a caregiver is, "Let me know if there is anything I can do or let me know if you need something." Let's be honest, most caregivers won't ask. Would you, when that person hasn't really been there for you during the caregiving process? Instead say something like, "I want to bring over a meal. When is a good day for you?" or "I would like to take your husband out for lunch to give you a break. What works for you?"

What is the best/worst thing you have learned about yourself? I have learned that I can do just about anything! Even when I think I can't go on anymore, I have found a way to keep going. I have endured way more than I thought possible. I'm stronger than I ever thought I could be.

What would you most like to tell someone who has become a caregiver? That the first year is a "hair on fire" kind of year. Learn all you can about what your significant other has been diagnosed with and become their advocate. If you don't, who will?

What would you do if someone handed you $100,000? I would use that money to make my husband's quality of life as good as humanly possible. That amount of money would allow me to hire people to come in our home and be able to keep him at home as long as possible. I would put a little of it away to help cover final expenses and maybe a vacation down the road for me.

What would you do with three extra hours a day? I would use that time to grocery shop, clean the house, and get out by myself. I would go see a movie or go to lunch. I don't really get any time to myself these days. At work my students always need me for something and at home my husband always needs me for something. It can get really overwhelming!

What do you wish you had more of? More time before this all started! I was only 45; he was only 57 when we started seeking help for his symptoms. Things started probably two years before that. We had been married for twenty years when his FTD symptoms became too much to ignore. I wish I had twenty more years before this happened to him.

What are some easy things you do to relax or find joy?

1. Talk to and spend time with my kids. They bring me the greatest joy right now.

2. Take a soak in the bathtub. This gives me a little alone time.

3. Go for a walk. This is my time to reflect and remember my purpose in life.

4. Put on my headphones and zone out to music or watch something on Netflix.

What are three things someone could do to help YOU (not your loved one, but you)?

1. Stay with him so I can have some time to myself. No one ever offers or asks if they can do something like that.

2. Be sincere when they ask how things are going. I feel like most people ask because it's what they think they should do. I feel they don't want to hear the real answer and/or don't know how to react if I tell them the truth.

3. Ask us to do things as a couple. That way it's not just me taking him places. It's lonely to go out to eat and not have a conversation during your meal or on the drive to get there.

When was the last time you cried? Yesterday; I was watching a TV show where three teenagers' dad died. It made me think about what's to come and how my kids will be affected even though they are in their 20s. Honestly, it seems like I cry almost every week about something, but then again, I am an emotional person.

Do you like yourself? Yes, I do. Am I perfect? Absolutely not! But I like the person I am and realize I have shortcomings. I try to be the best wife/mother/sister/friend that I can be.

What is the hardest thing you have faced? The uncertainty is one of the hardest things about this disease. There are constantly changing behaviors and there is no definitive progression or timeline. We are 7 ½ years in and really have no idea of what is yet to come. It could be one year, or it could be ten years. It makes it extremely difficult to plan for anything really.

What is the one thing that no one can understand about your situation? Plain and simple, what it's like to watch your husband die while he is still alive. He is not the same person I married. People with FTD go through personality changes. They lose their ability to do things the rest of us take for granted. No one can understand any of this unless they have lived through it.

Do you have support from family? Friends? Church? Others? My parents have been a great help. My husband worked for my family on the farm. My dad and brother were extremely good to him when he couldn't work full-time anymore. I have a couple of close friends that have provided me support as well.

What do you miss the most? I miss having a normal conversation and a physical and emotional connection with my husband. Being a caregiver for someone with FTD is a very lonely and heartbreaking journey.

List any resources that you have found helpful in your journey.

The private online support group for spouses of FTD has been the most helpful resource I've come across. Also, The Association for Frontotemporal Dementia (www.theaftd.org) is a great resource with tons of information and support.

CHRIS
Rio Grande, NJ

"We belong to a rare group who are heroes."

Caree and age at diagnosis: Joe, 57
Diagnosis: FTD, June 2015

Where do you find hope? Comfort? I found hope and comfort through Facebook support groups where I was able to read what other caregivers were going through and learned what was truly ahead of me. People who could literally say, "I know what you are going through; I can relate with you." That was comfort! I am not alone!

What is one thing about caregiving (or you or others) that surprised you most? I couldn't believe I could be a good caregiver. At first, I was bad at it, but I caught on after I educated myself. It's not easy going through the stages of grief while conquering the new caregiver role. I had to fight through the tears just to make it through the day. Understanding, empathy, and much more!

How do you take care of yourself? I had two choices: Go down with my husband as this disease took him down or stand up fight and do ME! I am too young to have my soul die. So, I get dressed and think about me too! In-home caregivers and nursing homes are needed to help me with this major task of caregiving. Girls' night out, spa days, shopping, etc.

What do you do when you hit bottom? I cry, feel like dying myself at times, get very depressed, and oh, so sad. Guilt settles in and I feel awful! WHY? I start praying, have faith in God, and get over it as quick as I can.

What is the best/worst piece of advice you have ever been given? I hate when people think my husband can be healed – "Have faith, there are miracles!" Yes, perhaps, but not for this awful brain disease, unfortunately. No hope here.

What is the best/worst thing you have learned about yourself? I am stronger than I ever thought I was. I am determined not to be defeated like my husband is being with this brain disease. I am a survivor and I have a job to do for my husband, my kids, and myself.

What would you most like to tell someone who has become a caregiver? Welcome to the world of crazy; nothing normal here. Have patience, educate yourself, understand the disease, and know what to expect. Don't forget about YOU. Treat yourself well. Don't let this disease bring you down into the dark tunnel. Being a caregiver is a heroic job. You are extremely special because you are a caregiver. Join others with whom you have this in common, learn from each other and support each other!

What would you do with three extra hours a day? SLEEP, SNORE, DREAM.

What do you wish you had more of? MONEY, of course! Good ole times with my honey. Laughter, love, and peace!

What are some easy things you do to relax or find joy? Read, go to the beach, bike ride, exercise, shop.

What is the best/worst question you have ever been asked? [Best:] To be on the panel for early onset caregivers by the Alzheimer's organization. To be hired as a patient care coordinator by our neurologist for his dementia center where I help others like myself. The nursing home staff and hospice nurse asking, "How can we help your husband? What does he like?"

What are three things someone could do to help YOU (not your loved one, but you)? CARE, show concern, support me!

When was the last time you cried? Five minutes ago. I do this at least every day more than once!

Do you like yourself? YES, of course I do. Sometimes conceited.

What is the hardest thing you have faced? Accepting and watching my husband die of frontotemporal disease.

What is the one thing that no one can understand about your situation? The need to be loved, have someone to talk to, make me feel special etc. Having a partner when I am still married.

What is it that everyone should know, but no one wants to talk about? What it feels like to lose your husband mentally after over thirty years of marriage. How am I still functioning? Why I do what I do and feel how I feel.

Do you have support from family? Friends? Church? Others? My family and friends only.

What do you miss the most? My relationship with my husband, my partner, my friend, my lover, my man. I miss his touch, his voice, the man he was, and everything he did for me. The smile he put on my face, his stories, and so much more.

Do you have a humorous story you would like to share? My husband did some wacky things before and after diagnosis. But before then, we used to ride bikes on the boardwalk in the morning, have breakfast, and ride again. We spent lots of time together where smiles and laughter were always a big part of the day!

Anything else you would like to add? Dementia hurts us more than it hurts our loved ones. It saddens us more and it kills us before it does them. We are special people, we belong to a rare group who are heroes; we are better than the doctors and nurses. We are in it because of love, devotion, and dedication. We are in it mind, body, and soul!

List any resources that you have found helpful in your journey.

I have so many resources from my community, but the best ones of all are the Alzheimer's Association website and The Association of Frontotemporal Degeneration website.

LEE
Discovery Bay, CA

"Try not to beat yourself up."

Caree and age at diagnosis: Scott, 53
Diagnosis: bvFTD, December 10, 2014

Where do you find hope? Comfort? I find hope in many ways. First of all, in educating myself in the disease. UCSF and its support staff have been a great source of information and comfort. I also attend a monthly support group at a local memory care facility. Most of all from the love of my family, my parents, his parents, our children and their families, best friends, and caring coworkers.

What is one thing about caregiving (or you or others) that surprised you most? As women we've spent our lives caring for spouse and children with physical illnesses, from colds to cancer. But a mental illness or impairment is so different. I was not prepared for it. I feel that I was not good at it. Even though family said I had the patience of a saint, inside I didn't feel that way at all because I know what was in my thoughts. The anguish and sense of failure.

How do you take care of yourself? I still work, so the "escape" to work and the distraction of my coworkers was an eight-hour break every day, even though it was often interrupted with calls of my husband falling and hurting himself. While my husband was still living at home, I was not taking care of myself, not seeing doctors regularly, like getting mammograms, dentist, and eye exams. They had little importance compared to what my husband was facing. And it was mentally very difficult.

What do you do when you hit bottom? Cried. Screamed. Often asking God, "Why?" I was a mess prior to having to place him in the care home. People with FTD can be so destructive, and even though I tried not to let the value of damaged and broken things or the destruction of the floors and rugs from getting peed on get to me, that those are material things, the daunting task of fixing and repairing fell now on my shoulders, when prior to the disease, it would have been my husband fixing everything. One day when he peed on my leg and then pooped in the shower, and the caregiver told me she couldn't handle him anymore…that was when I hit rock bottom and knew I couldn't do it anymore. Then the challenge of remodeling my home to accommodate him or place him came next.

What is the best/worst piece of advice you have ever been given? Seek help when you find yourself screaming and losing your mind. Don't feel like a failure when you have to place your loved one.

(I have a dear coworker whose mother had died of dementia. She gave me the book *The 36 Hour Day* as soon as she heard about my husband's diagnosis.) Everything in that book is valuable. Worst: constantly being told "Be sure to take care of yourself." They don't understand what it's like. How do you truly take care of yourself when you're giving all of yourself to caring for a person in the throes of FTD? It's extremely difficult. I can't imagine how people who do not work and have that time away from home, are able to do it.

What is the best/worst thing you have learned about yourself? That I'm resilient. That I can live through a lot of horrible things. That with a lot of thought and some experimentation, I can make some very good decisions. Worst, I still feel like I was not a good caregiver, not cut out for it.

What would you most like to tell someone who has become a caregiver? Hang in there, read *The 36 Hour Day*; read other suggested books from the FTD organization website; find a good medical resource to help you understand the disease and to help medicate your loved one. And if you find that you can't do it, that you're not cut out for it, try not to beat yourself up about it.

What would you do if someone handed you $100,000? I would have spent it to remodel my two-story house so that my husband would have had a downstairs room to be able to stay at home, and I'd have hired 24/7 caregivers just so that he could be at his home; and, give the rest to FTD research. (But now, looking back, I spent $102,500 in 18 months on care home costs alone, not including medication and supplies like diapers and wipes.) (And thank goodness for Blue Cross, because his hospital bill for infected bed sores was over $300,000 for an eleven-day stay.)

What would you do with three extra hours a day? Go outside and breathe. Read a book undisturbed. Nap.

What do you wish you had more of? Patience.

What are some easy things you do to relax or find joy? Visit family. Read. Sleep. Escape to the outdoors. Listen to music.

What is the best/worst question you have ever been asked? Worst: "You'll be happy when he dies, right?"

What are three things someone could do to help YOU (not your loved one, but you)? 1) Come help clean my house because I don't have the time or energy to do it. 2) Take me somewhere away from it all for a few hours.

When was the last time you cried? A couple of hours ago. My husband died on January 3, 2018. I just got an amazing letter from a retired coworker and it was so sweet and full of wonderful advice, I sobbed. Her husband died of Alzheimer's a few years ago, so she understands.

Do you like yourself? Yes, but I feel selfish because I did "think of myself" and did my best to do things to make myself happy.

What is the hardest thing you have faced? Chronologically, first was placing him in memory care; next was his death.

What is the one thing that no one can understand about your situation? The guilt of not being able to help him, even though we know the truth of the disease and its outcome. The feeling of being a failure.

What is it that everyone should know, but no one wants to talk about? That if you can place your loved one, it's heartbreaking but it will save your life. And also, some of the things our loved ones go through, like the amped up sex drive issues; and pooping! He smeared poop all over the bathroom while I slept one night. Horrible. The anger and disgust that comes from what we have to face is painful. As women, we think that we should be able to get past those things and put on a happy face.

Do you have support from family? Friends? Church? Others? I had family to talk to but no relief of my duties from them. When my husband was in board and care, my brother-in-law did volunteer to check on my husband so that I could take a vacation to visit my cousins. I must tell you here that two of his brothers did tell me that they would relieve me for a day if I wanted to go to a movie or something. They did keep an eye on him at a family party so that I could mingle and talk with people…very nice.

What do you miss the most? Kisses. Hugs. Conversations. Reassurance that my husband was there for me. Someone to go home to.

Do you have a humorous story you would like to share? It broke my heart to put my husband in memory care. I'd sit on the edge of my bed sleepless and crying at night, thinking that he was lonely too. About ten days after he'd been there the director of the facility saw me walking in from the parking lot and hurried outside to meet me. He said, "Lee, I need to talk to you. I'm not sure how to approach you about this. Sometimes when people in your husband's condition come to live in our facility, they strike up friendships, and sometimes they get very serious." I began laughing; I knew what he was going to say. I said, "Are you telling me that Scott has a girlfriend?" The director said that he couldn't believe that I was taking it so well. I told him the story of a family friend whose father had Alzheimer's. My friend would pick up his mom on Friday night, then go get dad at the care home to take him to dinner. One evening Henry Sr. asked if he could "bring his girlfriend along." So, I'd heard about this years ago and I was not surprised. I was actually relieved that he was not lonely.

Anything else you would like to add? Now let me add to the other side of my humorous story. Yes, I was relieved to see that Scott was not lonely, having his lady friend and all. But she was quite different than he was. Scott was nearly silent, rarely saying anything, or mumbling so that you could not understand him. She was vocal and the most uncooperative patient at the facility. One day, as I entered the locked facility, Scott happened to walk out of the recreation room. He saw me and walked straight towards me and as he approached he said, "I missed you." This was amazing; he had not spoken anything like that in months! But on his tail came the girlfriend. Scott turned to see her as she walked up to us. They kissed! Right in front of me! After he said he missed me! The workers started apologizing to me immediately, "Lee, we're sure he doesn't know what he's doing, he doesn't mean it." Even though I knew he'd lost his mind, it was still a stab in my heart. I said that I guess he didn't need me and asked to be let outside. I walked away with tears in my eyes. There were other odd moments like that. My husband fell constantly, having lost his sense of body placement. One afternoon when returning from the ER with fresh stitches in his head, I was happy that they had saved a lunch for him. We sat down alone in the dining room. The girlfriend noticed us and walked up. I figured what the heck and offered her a seat at the table. She down with us. I tried to strike up a friendly conversation and told her about his fall and showed her his stitches. She said to me, "You can leave now." I decided to remind her that I'm his wife and would sit with him while he ate his lunch. She said, "Well, you're never here!" Ouch, that one hurt again. But I kept my big girl face on and ignored it, but yes, I still feel the pain of her remark more than a year later.

List any resources that you have found helpful in your journey.
The memory care support group. Even if your loved one doesn't live there you are welcome to attend. I found that if you feel free to tell

others what you're going through, you will find many other who have also experienced it and are willing to talk. A local non-profit group called Care Quest helped with finding care facilities, calling ahead to see where there were vacancies and then giving me information and their care prices. FaceBook: there are several great groups, most of them closed so that outsiders don't see your comments and questions; groups such as "Memory People", "The FTD Spouse", "Caring for a Spouse with Dementia" and many others, including after the worst happens, "FTD Survivors – the Next Chapter" for loved ones of those who have died of FTD. Search key words in FB and you will find many caring groups.

SHELLI
Bakersfield, CA

"I'm still so lonely."

Caree and age at diagnosis: John, 45
Diagnosis: FTD, early 2015

Where do you find hope? Comfort? I find both hope and comfort in my children, parents, and wonderful friends.

What is one thing about caregiving (or you or others) that surprised you most? When we first began this journey, I felt strong and thought I would have no problem caring for my husband at home until the end. As the end becomes nearer, I am physically and mentally exhausted. Definitely not as easy as I had pictured in my head when he was still mobile.

How do you take care of yourself? Honestly, I don't. I haven't had my hair cut in two years. I have broken teeth that I tell myself I'll take care of when this journey is over. Sometimes I only get to shower once a week. At times, even longer. I feel guilty leaving him just so I can go to the grocery store.

What do you do when you hit bottom? Cry it out, remind myself that I'm going to see this through and that I CAN do it because I've come this far. In the beginning, I cried and cried and didn't think I was going to be capable of everything.

What is the best/worst piece of advice you have ever been given? To accept help when it is offered. To stop trying to do everything by myself.

What is the best/worst thing you have learned about yourself? The best thing I have learned…how STRONG I am.

What would you most like to tell someone who has become a caregiver? Pick your battles. Don't sweat the small stuff. The housework and dishes will be there tomorrow. Don't be afraid to ask for help and don't be too proud to accept help. One day at a time.

What would you do if someone handed you $100,000? Buy myself a car and a house for stability. Pay for my youngest two to finish college. Make a donation to AFTD. Save the rest for a rainy day.

What would you do with three extra hours a day? Make appointments for all of the dental work I need done, get my hair cut, go to a tanning booth, get a massage. All of that after I catch up on laundry and dishes and anything else that's been neglected in the house.

What do you wish you had more of? FTD is financially devastating, so I'm going to say money…so I could afford to have someone come and help me out during the day when I'm by myself with my husband.

What are some easy things you do to relax or find joy? Crossword puzzles. Watch "our shows" with my daughter on Tuesdays. Take in kitties that need to be bottle fed. Cuddle with my cats and listen to their relaxing purrs. Nap.

What is the best/worst question you have ever been asked? I honestly can't think of any best or worst questions. I welcome all questions because I take that opportunity to educate about FTD.

What are three things someone could do to help YOU (not your loved one, but you)? Help me with my laundry. Help me with my dishes. Send dinner.

When was the last time you cried? A few days ago. When I found out that a young (35) man in my town that had FTD passed away. He had two very young daughters and that just broke my heart.

Do you like yourself? Absolutely.

What is the hardest thing you have faced? The fact that my husband of 25 years will be going soon, along with any plans we had about retiring and spending the rest of our lives together doing fun things.

What is the one thing that no one can understand about your situation? That even though I'm surrounded by family and friends and people who love me…I'm still so lonely.

Do you have support from family? Friends? Church? Others? I am extremely fortunate to have a very supportive circle of family and friends. For that I feel truly blessed.

What do you miss the most? My best friend…my husband…his sense of humor, his smile, his smell…everything.

Anything else you would like to add? Frontotemporal dementia is a cruel and unforgiving disease. It can break the strongest person. I'm so grateful for the people I've met in my FTD support groups on Facebook. It really helps to know that you aren't alone in this nightmare and there is good advice to be found as well.

List any resources that you have found helpful in your journey. Theaftd.org has been the most helpful resource.

KATHY
Hiawatha, IA

"I cry often."

Caree and age at diagnosis: Tony, 45
Diagnosis: bvFTD, February 6, 2017

Where do you find hope? Comfort? Support of my friends, family, and community.

What is one thing about caregiving (or you or others) that surprised you most? I'm not sure it surprised me, but the rollercoaster. One minute I'm strong and able to do it, other times I feel weak and wonder how I will proceed. Somehow, some way I continue. You truly are stronger than you think, even when at times you don't think you are.

How do you take care of yourself? I take time for myself while I can. I accept help. I didn't at first, but I now allow people to take Tony for me, so I can have some time to get done what I need OR just read or catch up on sleep.

What do you do when you hit bottom? Call a friend and cry, stay in bed and allow myself to have a pity party if I find something for Tony to do. Mainly call family and friends for strength. I have to.

What is the best/worst thing you have learned about yourself? I'm so not patient, but I'm learning to be…it's taking time. I can be MEAN. There is always someone worse off in the world. The small things ARE SMALL. I now focus on what really matters. I don't sweat the small stuff.

What would you most like to tell someone who has become a caregiver? Patience isn't always inherited, it happens over time. You will become more patient than you ever knew you could be.

What would you do if someone handed you $100,000? Today: Invest it for future medical needs. 24-hour care. SAVE it and pretend I didn't have it OR pay for kids' college.

What would you do with three extra hours a day? Read a good book, take a nap, and watch TV with no interruption.

What do you wish you had more of? A clearer view of my future.

What are some easy things you do to relax or find joy? Exercise, take a nap, have lunch with friends, watch TV, and read.

What is the best/worst question you have ever been asked? "What did you do to piss off God?"

What are three things someone could do to help YOU (not your loved one, but you)? Do a budget for me. Help my kids get their college applications done. Put a roadmap together of what I need to be prepared for and how I will go about it.

When was the last time you cried? Two days ago. I cry often.

Do you like yourself? Yes, I am a kind, fun, and sweet person. I don't take care of myself though. I need to make better decisions with food (I use it as comfort).

What is the hardest thing you have faced? FTD – HANDS DOWN.

What is the one thing that no one can understand about your situation? A lot of it. The unknown future, the constant worry of "what's next." You can't turn your brain off completely and do the "take one day at a time." That's not reality. You have to be thinking ahead all the time.

Do you have support from family? Friends? Church? Others? Yes…all of the above. Thank goodness.

What do you miss the most? My best friend, my lover, my partner in crime, my one and only. The man I was supposed to grow old with. I miss the laughter, I miss sharing the responsibilities, I miss most how he would protect me and always have my back.

List any resources that you have found helpful in your journey.

The FTD Spouse on Facebook is a HUGE help and reading blogs caregivers write is helpful. The book *What If It's Not Alzheimer's?*

VICTORIA
Benson, NC

"What will happen to me after my husband is gone?"

Caree and age at diagnosis: Derek, 56
Diagnosis: bvFTD with PPA and generalized anxiety, April 1, 2016

Where do you find hope? Comfort? The FTD support group on Facebook, my two children, my friends, my grandchildren, and most important, my husband.

What is one thing about caregiving (or you or others) that surprised you most? It's a 24 hour, 7-days-a-week job. It can be lonely even with a great support team. The U.S. government is far behind in the needs of caregivers. If you don't plan early in your life, the cost of this disease is overwhelming. Especially since the primary age is 45 to 65. My husband was 56 when diagnosed. Two years after symptoms were showing themselves, we were not even thinking about retirement and now I ask myself, "If all our money is going to support my husband's care, what will happen to me after my husband is gone?" I am too young for Social Security, and who will hire anyone over age 55 in a job that will support me?

How do you take care of yourself? I have two caregivers come in two days a week for me to run the errands needed. I try and stay active and not think too much about my situation.

What do you do when you hit bottom? Cry and pray for guidance.

What is the best/worst piece of advice you have ever been given? Best advice: "One day at a time."

What is the best/worst thing you have learned about yourself? I try to control situations too much. Not too much surprises me anymore.

What would you most like to tell someone who has become a caregiver? Take it one day at a time. Gather your support team. Don't be surprised if a close family member is not part of that team. Keep your faith.

What would you do if someone handed you $100,000? Use it to make my husband as comfortable as possible with in-home care and companionship so I can get a part time job.

What would you do with three extra hours a day? Nothing. Not enough time is not a problem for me.

What do you wish you had more of? More time with my husband before the illness took him.

What are some easy things you do to relax or find joy? Play computer games, read, watch TV, shop, play with my grandchildren.

What is the best/worst question you have ever been asked? Best question: "Are you OK?" Worst question: "What are you going to do?"

What are three things someone could do to help YOU (not your loved one, but you)? Help me with the yard. Redo my bathroom to make it wheelchair accessible. Watch hubby while I take a day off.

When was the last time you cried? One week ago.

Do you like yourself? Yes.

What is the hardest thing you have faced? The loss of the man I married and the intimacy we shared. No more enjoying vacations together.

What is the one thing that no one can understand about your situation? At times I feel like my life is at a standstill. Until my husband passes away, I am not living life, I am existing. I am tired of taking care of someone who can't take care of themselves. And I am afraid to meet anyone else for fear I will have to take care of them.

What is it that everyone should know, but no one wants to talk about? Besides the loss of your best friend, who is replaced with a selfish stranger, you are still expected by outsiders to love them the same way.

Do you have support from family? Friends? Church? Others? Yes, all of the above.

What do you miss the most? Laughing with my husband, planning our future, enjoying life together, enjoying and planning vacations.

Do you have a humorous story you would like to share? Yes. In the beginning I was so bored, as hubby would sleep most of the time, that I invited the Kirby vacuum cleaner salesman to come inside and show me how his vacuum worked. I got to talk with someone and had my carpets cleaned. It was a very pleasant evening.

Anything else you would like to add? Taking a much-needed respite break in upstate NY with some of my family. Took a walk this morning and came across this road sign and wondered to myself "What's around the corner," and kept on walking. Once I got there, I found this hill and another curve in the road and for some reason, I just had to see what was around the second curve. So, I kept on walking and was focused on getting to the next curve to see what was there.

When I finally got there, I found another curve. My head said let's go to the next curve to see what's there, but my cold feet wanted to turn around and start walking back, which I did. While walking back, I realized, life is a lot like this road. You're going to have your ups and downs and there will be curves in your life. If you just focus on what is around the next curve, you're going to miss the beauty of life that's right in front of you and your support team that is always there waiting for you. Thank you, Dwight and Karen, for inviting me into your beautiful lake house. And Aunt Jean, thanks for always being on the front porch waiting for me. Life is beautiful, but you make it brighter.

List any resources that you have found helpful in your journey.
Facebook support groups.

ANONYMOUS
United Kingdom

"Give me some time home alone."

Caree and age at diagnosis: Spouse, 62
Diagnosis: bvFTD, September 21, 2017

Where do you find hope? Comfort? I'm not sure that I have any hope, or maybe I'm just having a bad day.
How do you take care of yourself? I get outside in the fresh air as much as possible.
What do you do when you hit bottom? Cry!
What is the best/worst thing you have learned about yourself? I don't have a great deal of patience, and mine is sorely tested at time.
What would you most like to tell someone who has become a caregiver? Look after yourself.
What would you do if someone handed you $100,000? Probably share it around a bit, give some to charity. I'm not motivated by money.
What would you do with three extra hours a day? Sleep.
What do you wish you had more of? Patience.
What are some easy things you do to relax or find joy? Listen to music. Walk the dog. Play the piano. Do some gardening. More gardening.
What is the best/worst question you have ever been asked? Worst – "Is he getting better?" No, what part of progressive, terminal illness do you not understand?
What are three things someone could do to help YOU (not your loved one, but you)? Give me some time home alone, i.e. take him out for a while. Just listen. Cook dinner.
When was the last time you cried? This morning.
Do you like yourself? Not a great deal.
What is the hardest thing you have faced? Death of my father.
What is the one thing that no one can understand about your situation? "That's just Kev, that's just the way he is." No, it's not. It's like my husband has been taken over by an alien and no one else can see it.
What is it that everyone should know, but no one wants to talk about? Your sex life will change, and not for the better.
Do you have support from family? Friends? Church? Others? Family and friends.
What do you miss the most? Having a companion, someone to talk to and share things with.

Do you have a humorous story you would like to share? Not at the moment.

MAGGIE
South Wales, UK

"Enjoy the time together."

Caree and age at diagnosis: Paul, 52
Diagnosis: bvFTD, February 2016

Where do you find hope? Comfort? I find hope in seeing online that my husband isn't as combative as others and is still fairly cooperative; and I find comfort in knowing that the community we live in is always looking out for us.

What is one thing about caregiving (or you or others) that surprised you most? That I have more patience than I thought possible.

How do you take care of yourself? I make sure I have "down time" at least once a week with friends to have a coffee; I also use working as a respite, too. Who knew!?

What do you do when you hit bottom? Eat more cake and chocolate, curse a lot, and take a long walk with our dog.

What is the best/worst piece of advice you have ever been given? Always take time for myself no matter what. I can't really say I've been given bad advice.

What is the best/worst thing you have learned about yourself? That I have more patience, but I have a bitch inside that wants to be cruel.

What would you most like to tell someone who has become a caregiver? That no matter how rubbish your day is, to enjoy the time together; and even though the person you're caring for may not realize it, their day is way worse! BUT, you're doing a great job regardless.

What would you do if someone handed you $100,000? Give half to research and take a blooming good holiday, then probably have to use the rest to pay for care.

What would you do with three extra hours a day? Pluck my eyebrows, shave my legs maybe, and catch up with much needed sleep!

What do you wish you had more of? Time before diagnosis.

What are some easy things you do to relax or find joy? Enjoy a cup of tea and a chocolate, listen to music whilst walking the dog, Sunday roast dinner with all the family, long hot shower, and my Saturday morning catch up with a friend.

What is the best/worst question you have ever been asked? Best: "How are YOU doing?" Worst: "What tablets are Paul on to get better?"!!!!

What are three things someone could do to help YOU (not your loved one, but you)? Keep the promises of, "Yes, I'll sit with him." Listen to me, and not think they know better and understand there are reasons I do the things I do, so don't undermine me and make me feel like rubbish.

When was the last time you cried? Today, every day, about something else Paul can no longer do.

Do you like yourself? Absolutely.

What is the hardest thing you have faced? Having to put our previous dog to sleep, without the support of Paul.

What is the one thing that no one can understand about your situation? The loneliness.

What is it that everyone should know, but no one wants to talk about? In my case, the massive change in personality, and you just have to suck it up, going from being wife/friend/lover into carer/nobody/slave.

Do you have support from family? Friends? Church? Others? I have great support from family and friends, I should let them do more; and also, we live in a wonderful community that always lets me know if Paul has wandered too far or is inappropriately dressed for the climate; and we get cakes etc. just when you need a pick-me-up. I don't go to church, but I do believe in God.

What do you miss the most? Too much to give one answer, it's just being a couple, doing regular things, having a drink (he's not allowed, so I can't either) but, if I had to pick one, going to the cinema. His toilet habits and lack of concentration would kill it for the whole audience.

Do you have a humorous story you would like to share? Again, too many, because you have to find humor in everything!

Anything else you would like to add? You're not alone on this hellish journey, take help whenever you can. Get both of you a social worker, and legal advice if necessary for your finances. Don't doubt your gut feelings, push for answers. Keep a journal, and remember, none of it is anything you've done. Stay strong.

TAMMY
Plymouth, IL

"I wish there was more of me."

Caree and age at diagnosis: Gregg, 59
Diagnosis: bvFTD, March 2017

Where do you find hope? Comfort? Hope, I hope that he can hold on for at least five years. It will give him more time to watch the grandchildren grow. They are 3 and 6 now and learning and growing so fast. Comfort? I find comfort in my family, our church family, and GOD.

What is one thing about caregiving (or you or others) that surprised you most? Many things surprised me. When I told his family, I received many different comments. Ranging from "That's too bad." "How do you know? Did you go to the doctor or do you just think he has FTD?" to "Well, don't worry, he can beat it."

How do you take care of yourself? I don't! That's the problem. At times I feel the world of FTD is trying to swallow me whole. Finally, I went to therapy, put on three types of blood pressure meds (once it reached 190/105, I became scared for my own life).

What do you do when you hit bottom? I tell him to give me 30 minutes. I go take a hot shower and cry. That steam soothes my tense muscles, and the crying relieves the internal pressure causing me to be mad, and/or sad. It's like steam from a teapot, it relieves pressure.

What is the best/worst piece of advice you have ever been given? The worst, "It's his disease, he doesn't know what he is saying." "You wouldn't argue with a drunk, so don't argue with him. He can't be reasoned with."

What is the best/worst thing you have learned about yourself? I have realized that I am a strong woman, and that we are blessed by having strong children. I heard this saying one day…We are only as strong as the strength of our family. The worst: That the love for my husband has changed. I still love him, but not in love. The fall out of FTD just killed off the love. I wasn't able to press back the changes happening to him and our family.

What would you most like to tell someone who has become a caregiver? You and only YOU know your limits and those of the one with FTD. When people offer stupid advice and trust me you will receive a lot…. I will have to think about that, thank you for giving me that idea.

What would you do if someone handed you $100,000? Cry with relief knowing that I now have the funds to keep my loved one comfortable and safe. Also, like anyone else, I would pay off all our bills, and pay all the student loans our children have incurred for college. Donate a chunk for research so just maybe another family can be spared from this nightmare.

What would you do with three extra hours a day? Go shopping for groceries by myself. Take a nice long bath and either a nap or curl up with a good book.

What do you wish you had more of? I wish there was more of me. I wish I had more patience, and on certain days I wish I had more grace.

What are some easy things you do to relax or find joy? To be able to call my mother. To just sit and gossip. Talking to our children either via phone, text, or Facebook. Most of all is being able to talk to our 3- and 6-year-old granddaughters via Facetime. But mostly to be able to just go and sit in the sanctuary of our little country church. I sit and talk to God and when I am done, I just keep sitting there letting the peace permeate my soul.

What is the best/worst question you have ever been asked? The only question that has been continuously asked is, "How is Gregg?" Would they want to hear about how he can't pee in the toilet when the floor seems a better choice to him? I think not. The best for me is the simple, "I am thinking of you, please call me if you need anything," followed by a hug. It's a very lonely time. Just knowing you aren't alone is worth a lot.

What are three things someone could do to help YOU (not your loved one, but you)? Offer to help me at home. Do the stuff that bothers me, but I don't have the time or drive to accomplish. Spend the day at my house, talk, laugh, and joke while we clean baseboards, clean out closets, paint the inside of said closet.

When was the last time you cried? About a month ago: When I was pulling into the driveway to find him pulling my old couch out of the house and putting it on the wagon. He was tired of looking at it. I cried for days. Yes, it was old, but I threw a quilt over it. Cried wondering where the money would come to buy a new one.

Do you like yourself? This is a two-sided coin. I like the inside me. I am loving, care for others, always willing to help. I dislike (bordering along hate) the outside of me. I need a haircut, and the gray hair is taking over. I am 35 pounds overweight, and I have bags under my eyes from being perpetually tired.

What is the hardest thing you have faced? That my loving husband is/has disappeared in front of me. That our hopes and dreams are either gone or greatly altered.

What is the one thing that no one can understand about your situation? How lonely, isolated you feel along with the grieving that starts before your loved one has passed from this life.

What is it that everyone should know, but no one wants to talk about? The fight that you have to face and endure so that FTD doesn't steal your compassion, your joy, your sense of worth. That it doesn't steal your soul. The fight is real.

Do you have support from family? Friends? Church? Others? My children, daughter-in-law and son-in-law are my rock. My granddaughters are the soft place I can land. My church family is always there at the waiting to help.

What do you miss the most? The years when we were a young family. The joy he found being outside with the kids riding motorcycles and four-wheelers. But most of all, the times he would tell them, "You need to go to college, I want a better life for you." Our children miss the hugs and him saying, "I love you," at the end of their phone calls.

Do you have a humorous story you would like to share? Unfortunately, no! With bvFTD, the laughter and joy go away. Left behind in its wake.

Anything else you would like to add? If you should live in a rural community as I do, please don't become discouraged. People believe FTD is just like Alzheimer's. Only we know it's different. If you are at the beginning of the journey, find a support group. Even if the only choice is an Alzheimer's group. I was able to take away many techniques to help deal with this horrendous journey.

LINDA
Lexington, KY

"Don't think too far ahead."

Caree and age at diagnosis: Kenny, 62
Diagnosis: FTD, April 2014; ALS, October 2016

Where do you find hope? Comfort? I take a day at a time and try not to think too far ahead so I don't get overwhelmed and feel hopeless. I find comfort from the caring I have received from friends, neighbors, and family.

What is one thing about caregiving (or you or others) that surprised you most? The main thing I am surprised about is how good I am at it and how strong of a woman I really am.

How do you take care of yourself? I work out at the gym and I take a night or day when I feel I need it.

What do you do when you hit bottom? I think this won't be forever and I am luckier than a lot of people in my same situation.

What is the best/worst piece of advice you have ever been given? Best advice was to get control of the finances. Worst advice was to get marriage counseling.

What is the best/worst thing you have learned about yourself? The best is how strong I am. I don't feel like there isn't anything I can't do. The worst thing I've learned is I wasted a lot of years being mad about stupid stuff and worrying about things that really don't matter.

What would you most like to tell someone who has become a caregiver? Take one day at a time and don't think too far ahead or you will drive yourself crazy. You will find out who really cares about you and don't waste time being mad at the ones who don't. Move on.

What would you do if someone handed you $100,000? I would probably put it away for when needed. But I would spend some on myself, like a trip. I would use on respite care, but mainly save for down the road when I will need help in caring for him, like bathing, etc.

What would you do with three extra hours a day? Sleep.

What do you wish you had more of? I wish my family lived closer to me.

What are some easy things you do to relax or find joy? Work out and yoga. Talk and drink wine with friends. Watch TV. Go to University of Kentucky men's basketball games. Go see my great niece and nephew twins who are 18 months old and just so adorable.

What is the best/worst question you have ever been asked? Best: "I really want to help you, what can I do?" Worst: "Are you taking care of yourself? You need to take care of yourself."

What are three things someone could do to help YOU (not your loved one, but you)? Yard work. Take him so I could have time alone. Yard work.

When was the last time you cried? I can't remember. I can't cry anymore.

Do you like yourself? Yes, more than ever.

What is the hardest thing you have faced? I would say this is (husband's FTD). The hardest part of that was the beginning and finding out the financial destruction and dealing with all his business stuff all alone.

What is the one thing that no one can understand about your situation? I don't think anyone could understand anything about this if it's not happening or has happened to them. It's too bizarre to try to even explain.

What is it that everyone should know, but no one wants to talk about? I can't think of anything I don't talk with people about.

Do you have support from family? Friends? Church? Others? Friends, family, neighbors.

What do you miss the most? I miss having my husband for advice and the freedom to go and do whatever I want whenever I want.

List any resources that you have found helpful in your journey.

My older sister – her husband had FTD and died. FTD Facebook Spouse group. The internet.

ANONYMOUS
Washington

"Be grateful for what is given."

Caree and age at diagnosis: Spouse, 62
Diagnosis: FTD, June 2016

Where do you find hope? Comfort? I believe in a G-d who is sovereign, in all things, even the hard ones, and that He is the only wise G-d who is working His plan out in every moment. He knows the number of our days and has purpose for us in living them. He has surrounded me with friends and a faith community who are praying and encouraging us often.

What is one thing about caregiving (or you or others) that surprised you most? How quickly this could progress (in our case). When I realized that FTD was what my husband had (prior to seeing the doctor), I wrote in a journal my hope and plan for walking through this with him in a way that honored G-d. The first thing that came to my mind was the words to an old, old hymn, "Whate'er My G-d Ordains Is Right." I wasn't prepared for how often I'd feel blown off course by circumstances and how difficult it would be (in my own strength) to get back on course. This is no surprise, but I believe this is as much about what G-d wants to do to refine me as it is about my husband.

How do you take care of yourself? I walk with one of my closest friends five mornings a week. She is a recent widow whose husband died from a brain tumor (temporal) after only four months, and she understands much of what we are going through. I'm very grateful for her friendship and presence in my life and that we can share this journey of processing losses together.

What do you do when you hit bottom? Retreat to a spare bedroom upstairs alone (my "office" with a sunny window) and regroup, looking ahead to the next alone-time, sometimes writing a list of things I need to work on during that time. Read a short piece I put together after reading *Holding Space*.

What is the best/worst piece of advice you have ever been given? Best: Try to grasp the losses as they come rather than gunny-sacking them for later. Worst: People have been very kind and generally very careful in what they've said. There are several who have "suggested" they believe my husband's condition could be reversed with the avoidance of certain foods and the addition of particular supplements…The reality is that there's only so much you can control, and that food and fellowship go together…and fellowship is so important. So, we do what we can at home and let the rest go. His happiness is important.

What is the best/worst thing you have learned about yourself? That I'm very capable of behaving badly...becoming angry and losing my temper with him, shaming him, showing him my frustration, making him feel inadequate, etc., and it can easily become habitual. Also, [caregiving] cannot be done in my own strength.

What would you do if someone handed you $100,000? At first, I saw "1 thousand dollars"—100 thousand changes it! I might actually look for some paid outside help at this point. He is bored to death. He can no longer comprehend, but he "reads" the same books over and over again, "watches" NCIS on his iPad (though that's suddenly happening less this week). Listening to audio books doesn't work. He can no longer play a simple game of dominoes or put together a child's jigsaw puzzle. He can and does split wood on occasion but is done after two pieces. He can't complete a task, and I'm at a loss for finding something that he enjoys enough to stick with it for more than a couple of minutes. A consultant would be a good investment! Also, I know he'd enjoy a week in Hawaii's warm water.

What would you do with three extra hours a day? I might get food prep done so that I could be free to sit with him more. (I know that's not technically a "good" answer.) I might read and write (journal), or work on some creative pursuits.

What do you wish you had more of? Time alone. Before his diagnosis, I was used to over eleven hours a day on my own. I worked part time, but still had plenty of time to read, create, spend time with a friend from time to time, just BE.

What are some easy things you do to relax or find joy? Read, garden (get dirt under my fingernails!), play the piano, drink a cup of coffee, plan a project. Walk through Hobby Lobby—alone. Go to the library—alone.

What are three things someone could do to help YOU (not your loved one, but you)? Take my husband somewhere on a drive—do anything with him, without me. (That WOULD be for me!) Go to dinner with us. Conversation, no meal prep/serving/clean up. Help me with tech questions—He was a Systems Engineer but is completely baffled by technology now.

When was the last time you cried? I'm not a crier, but I do "leak" from time to time. Yesterday we walked to our town's sweet little coffee shop for a cup of coffee and a scone. Don't often do it, so it was a treat for me. No conversation, scone wolfed staring straight ahead so he dropped a lot, coffee swallowed as quickly as possible, and ready to go. It made me very sad. We used to love to eat out—a lot—and he always had very good table manners. But…the gist of the words I heard Elizabeth Elliott say over forty years ago (I can't find the exact quote as I remember it) came back to me as we walked home: "Be grateful for what is given rather than resentful over what is withheld."

Do you like yourself? Not a lot of the time.

What is the hardest thing you have faced? So far, I can't complain a lot. His obsessive-compulsive behaviors bother me a lot and make me uncomfortable in social situations, though our friends and family understand. (The compulsive eating is particularly hard.) And there's his lack of insight into his behaviors. (Gee, thanks for asking THIS hard question! The following has been a good exercise. I've avoided working through this one) I think the one thing I am currently struggling with is my changing role with my husband. I didn't expect this, but I am at a place where I don't want to be intimate with him anymore, and, because of that, I don't touch him with affection fearing it will be misunderstood. At the same time, I know it is a basic human need. On the infrequent occasion he initiates, he uses the term "make love," but "have sex" would be more appropriate and while it's not at all unkind, it leaves me feeling very empty and objectified, I guess. It's another of those losses to grieve, but beyond that, I am his wife, and he is still my husband, and the L-rd has things to say about this. Does that change when someone has dementia?? I also read recently the quote from Shakespeare's Sonnet 116, "Love is not love which alters when it alteration finds," and wonder at its applicability.

What is the one thing that no one can understand about your situation? I'm not sure about this…

Do you have support from family? Friends? Church? Others? Yes – three of our four grown children (33-41), however, only one lives within 15 miles. The other two care and come when they can. We've traveled twice with one son and his family. We seem to be estranged from our other son who lives 300 miles away. His father and step mom are still alive—and in their 80s/90s—and live three hours away. We see them 4-5 times a year as well as his brother and wife. They love us, and I know they pray for us consistently. His mom was diagnosed with Alzheimer's at the age of 57 and died when she was 65. I wonder if it was really FTD. We have a very close faith "family" and the men he has been in relationship with and is still in a Bible study with are very considerate and patient with him now that he is different. One takes him for 4-6 hours once every four months or so to go to a museum, or to Cabela's and out to lunch. And old friends—from high school and young adulthood as well as from other states we've lived in—have returned into our lives (mine really) and are a source of encouragement. It has occurred to me that they are also "witnesses of my life."

What do you miss the most? Conversation and companionship over dinner, in the garden, on a drive, all the time. Someone to share the things that I'd only tell my husband. He was always my best friend—the one who knew me better than anyone else and still loved me. Being completely relaxed. This is an important one: The "witness to my life" – that's a term I've thought about a lot.

Anything else you would like to add? This is the reminder I wrote to myself after reading *Holding Space* by Heather Plett, "The ministry of presence is the willingness to walk alongside someone in whatever journey they are on with an open heart, gentle guidance when needed, humility and thoughtfulness, unconditional support and love without making them feel inadequate or shaming them, overwhelming them, or taking away their power giving them only as much as they can handle, making them feel safe even when they make mistakes or forget, are afraid, or fall apart. Be a refuge—a safe place—to express their emotions and fears."

List any resources that you have found helpful in your journey.
I found *What If It's Not Alzheimer's* on a display shelf at the library while I was combing through the shelves (pre-diagnosis) looking for what else his behavior could possibly be related to (Vitamin deficiency? Thyroid? Blood flow/something chiropractic could help?)—not expecting to find his exact symptoms described! So very thankful. I know this helped in obtaining an immediate diagnosis from his GP and then confirmed by the neurologist. (And this GP had seen FTD twice during his residency.) G-d's in the details! The HR representative at the company he was employed with who was willing to talk with me, suggest a course of action and offered hope. ("Don't wait! Go to a doctor, request a leave of absence to discover what's going on before he's let go!") He was placed on short-term disability immediately which, after six months, was converted to long-term disability for a total of five years' coverage. *Finding Grace in the Face of Dementia*, by John

Dunlop, MD. This is a book I'm slowly reading through and absorbing when I have an opportunity to be alone. It's written from the very perspective I want—one that honors G-d in this.

GINA
Orrstown, PA

"Make me feel like I'm special."

Caree and age at diagnosis: David, 43
Diagnosis: bvFTD with Semantic PPA, 2013

Where do you find hope? Comfort? Family, friends. Online support groups.

What is one thing about caregiving (or you or others) that surprised you most? Everyone says they will be there for you, but usually don't really mean it (or act on it).

How do you take care of yourself? Coffee. I go to college online to take my mind off of things.

What do you do when you hit bottom? Cry. Talk to my children. Hang out with cats and the dog.

What is the best/worst piece of advice you have ever been given? Don't be afraid to ask for help.

What is the best/worst thing you have learned about yourself? I should have divorced my husband years ago.

What would you most like to tell someone who has become a caregiver? Get support no matter what.

What would you do if someone handed you $100,000? Get a live-in caregiver.

What would you do with three extra hours a day? Sleep.

What do you wish you had more of? Patience.

What are some easy things you do to relax or find joy? Listen to music. Glass of wine/some kind of alcohol. Read. Cuddle with my kids/pets. Talk to my mom/friends.

What is the best/worst question you have ever been asked? "How do you deal with everything?"

What are three things someone could do to help YOU (not your loved one, but you)? Organize my house. Landscape. Make me feel like I'm special.

When was the last time you cried? Yesterday.

Do you like yourself? Sometimes.

What is the hardest thing you have faced? My son's incarceration and my husband's illness.

What is the one thing that no one can understand about your situation? How lonely it is.

What is it that everyone should know, but no one wants to talk about? Get a will/long-term care insurance.

Do you have support from family? Friends? Church? Others? Yes, but limited support.

What do you miss the most? Having someone to talk to and someone that cares about me.

List any resources that you have found helpful in your journey. Online support groups AFTD.

STEPHANIE
Dalton, MA

"I try to take time off each day."

Caree and age at diagnosis: Tom, 54
Diagnosis: FTD with MND, December 2016

Where do you find hope? Comfort? This is difficult to answer. I try to find my hope and comfort in the Lord. This is hard for me at times, so when I'm having a hard time, I call upon my friends; some are pastors, and some are lifelong friends. I enjoy going to my office in the morning when it is quiet, and I just sit in the comfort of just being alone with no distractions.

What is one thing about caregiving (or you or others) that surprised you most? The one thing that surprised me the most is having to do everything. No longer having a partner to share things with. On a positive note, this has made me a stronger and better person. I didn't know I had this much strength.

How do you take care of yourself? I try to take time off each day (doesn't always happen) to just do something for me. I started to go to a gym with a friend and I do line dancing when I find extra time. I also see a therapist every other week, this keeps me sane. At first, I didn't do anything for me, but you need to, it is very important.

What do you do when you hit bottom? The first thing I usually do is cry. A friend once told me that you need to cry at times, so you can release your emotions and give it to God. Then I usually call my dear friend who is a pastor. He is always there for me and knows how to lift me with his words and prayers. But I have to say, if you feel like crying, just do it, and don't hold back.

What is the best/worst piece of advice you have ever been given? The best advice is a few things: cry when you need to cry, make sure you take time each day for yourself, and to cherish each and every moment with your loved one as much as possible. Make memories that you will remember. The worst piece of advice is not so much advice as it is the words people say to you. This is what I always hear: "Tom looks great today, he must be getting better, I don't see anything wrong with him." Don't take this to heart as I sometimes do. You know your loved one and what he or she is going through, trust in your heart and mind.

What is the best/worst thing you have learned about yourself? The worst thing is that I am not always patient with my husband as I think I should be. I beat myself up all the time for not being patient.

The best thing is the strength I never knew I had until he got sick. I know in my heart I will be okay.

What would you most like to tell someone who has become a caregiver? Very important, take care of yourself first and foremost. We don't always do this. But if we are not healthy and happy, we can't take care of someone else. Take time for yourself as much as you can. Take help if it is offered, even if it is very hard for you, do it. And just make sure you continue to breathe each day.

What would you do if someone handed you $100,000? First thought is to run away, but that's not possible. I would first and foremost, to be honest, put some aside so that our daughter would always be taken care of. Then I would make sure it went to help caregivers, so that they can get the much-needed respite they need. I should say to put towards finding a cure for FTD, but there is not much out there for caregivers.

What would you do with three extra hours a day? Sleep and then watch a movie or go shopping all by myself. But first and foremost, would be sleep.

What do you wish you had more of? I wish I had more time with the husband I married, not the FTD husband.

What are some easy things you do to relax or find joy? Meditate, prayer, going to the gym, dance, and watch our daughter dance.

What is the best/worst question you have ever been asked? The worst question is, "How is Tom doing?" I don't think there has ever been a best question. I really hate when people ask how he is doing. He is dying a horrible death. "How do you think he is doing?" that's the answer I would like to give.

What are three things someone could do to help YOU (not your loved one, but you)? Listen to me when I am having a bad day. Make a meal or two so I don't have to. Send me flowers just to say I'm thinking about you.

When was the last time you cried? Last night while watching a show on TV.

Do you like yourself? Not always. I sometimes hate myself for the things I think and for the way I act. It is getting harder and harder for me to like myself.

What is the hardest thing you have faced? Honestly, it was the day we received the diagnosis. I'm sure there will be more, but right now this day. The day I saw my husband cry for the first time.

What is the one thing that no one can understand about your situation? How hard it is to watch your loved one suffer each and every minute of the day. He is no longer the man I married. This is not cancer, this is not a broken bone, this is a horrible disease that is killing his brain (who he is) and destroying his muscles.

What is it that everyone should know, but no one wants to talk about? How lonely we as caregivers are. And that just because our loved ones act normal when you see them, it is not how it is when they are home.

Do you have support from family? Friends? Church? Others? Yes, I have support from my family, not his. Our friends and church members are very supportive.

What do you miss the most? What I miss the most is my husband making love to me, holding my hand, kissing me, hugging me, and physical contact.

Do you have a humorous story you would like to share? My husband and I try to bring humor into our lives every day. I truly believe that if we didn't, we would both be in a worse place. When he is having a bad day with whatever it may be, I try to make a joke about it; he sometimes laughs. No real stories, just keep humor in your life.

Anything else you would like to add? Each and every person who has FTD is different from the next person; no two are alike. Both my husband's father and older brother died from a variation of this disease. My husband was never sick one day in his life, ever, until FTD struck him three years ago. Be honest with yourself, always. Cry when you need to cry, reach out when you need to, not when it's too late. Love your family always and try your hardest to be patient. You are not alone in this journey, whether you have faith or not, you do not walk this road alone.

List any resources that you have found helpful in your journey.

I have taken a caregiver's course with Home Instead, which has helped a lot. I also attend a support group once a month with [Home Instead] for caregivers. The FTD support group on Facebook helps.

MARY
Two Rivers, WI

"Some days life just gets to be too much."

Caree and age at diagnosis: William, 59
Diagnosis: bvFTD, October 2015

Where do you find hope? Comfort? Facebook – The FTD Spouse page. I have found this the best source of information and comfort because they understand what I am going through.

How do you take care of yourself? I read, knit, crochet. I ride my motorcycle in the summer time. I get a massage every now and then.

What is the best/worst piece of advice you have ever been given? The worst was someone suggested that my husband might have Lyme Disease. The best was when I was trying to get my husband to eat at an earlier time at night, and he refused. I was told to just deal with it, I can't reason with someone whose 'reasoner' was broken.

What is the best/worst thing you have learned about yourself? The best is that I am a strong person. The worst is that I realized that I am only human and that some days life just gets to be too much.

What would you most like to tell someone who has become a caregiver? Being a caregiver isn't for everyone. Some people just can't handle it. That is when you need to let someone else do the caregiving.

What would you do if someone handed you $100,000? I would take a vacation by myself and I would put the rest in the bank and spend it wisely.

What would you do with three extra hours a day? My husband goes to day care four to five hours a day. If I had an extra three hours, I would take a nap.

What do you wish you had more of? Hours in a day. Even though my husband goes to day care four to five hours, it seems there is never enough time in a day to do the things I want to get done. But there is always tomorrow.

What are some easy things you do to relax or find joy? Ride my motorcycle in the summer, knit, crochet, read, get a massage.

What are three things someone could do to help YOU (not your loved one, but you)? Help me do a thorough cleaning of my house, thorough cleanup of my yard, buy me a car that won't nickel and dime me.

When was the last time you cried? A few weeks ago.

Do you like yourself? Yes

What is the hardest thing you have faced? Having to be a caregiver to my husband. I took care of other members of his family in different capacities. My husband having bvFTD is the hardest seeing him disappear into someone I don't know.

What is the one thing that no one can understand about your situation? How really hard it is to be a caregiver of someone with dementia. Listening to the repetitive questions or listening to the repetitive statements.

What is it that everyone should know, but no one wants to talk about? That my husband will die from this disease.

Do you have support from family? Friends? Church? Others? I have emotional support from my family. His family calls only once in a while. The most support I get is from our Harley friends.

What do you miss the most? My husband. Being able to go places and do things, i.e. vacations.

List any resources that you have found helpful in your journey.

Facebook – The FTD Spouse page. (Local agencies had nothing on this disease.) I would be going nuts without them.

ELAINE
Federal Way, WA

"For now, he needs me."

Caree and age at diagnosis: Herbert, 65
Diagnosis: FTD/PPA, 2014

Where do you find hope? Comfort? There is no hope. I find comfort in God and my family…and my memories. My son and daughter are living with us, and they're here to offer help if I need it and if they're able.

What is one thing about caregiving (or you or others) that surprised you most? How difficult it is to get help. The VA said they could send someone twice a week, but now that we're at the point that I could use someone, I'm told that funding was cut back in 2015. Dead end…

How do you take care of yourself? I've loaded my home with craft supplies, two rescue dogs, and two cockatoos, so no time to be bored. My family loves my Herb as much as I do, and they stop by for a visit as often as they can. I really depend on them for moral support.

What do you do when you hit bottom? I don't think I've hit there yet. I know we have a long way to go and I don't want to darken the time we have left thinking about it. I try to be positive for him. There will be time to cry later. For now, he needs me.

What is the best/worst piece of advice you have ever been given? To keep in mind that they can't help or control the way they are or the things they do or won't do. The negative stuff is the disease, not something they're doing intentionally. And let them know how much you love them…always.

What is the best/worst thing you have learned about yourself? I've learned that God must have a lot of faith in me to have entrusted me with this job. I've learned also that I need to dig deep to find that faith in myself so that the fear and dread of what's to come doesn't overwhelm me. I'm finding I'm stronger than I thought possible when I need to be.

What would you most like to tell someone who has become a caregiver? Love them. They're so lost and afraid and need our love so badly. Also, line up help before you need it.

What would you do if someone handed you $100,000? I'd renovate our home to make it wheelchair accessible before we get to that point, and to hire the help I need for a few hours a week, so I could take an art class or do the grocery shopping without having to worry about him.

What would you do with three extra hours a day? I'd spend half on myself and half cuddling with my Herb.

What do you wish you had more of? Knowledge of how to find the resources we need and where to learn to better my skills of caregiving.

What are some easy things you do to relax or find joy? 1. Spend time with my kids or grandkids. 2. Cuddle my dogs. 3. Play with my birds. 4. Work on a craft project. 5. Read a book.

What is the best/worst question you have ever been asked? I was asked why he won't just snap out of it.

What are three things someone could do to help YOU (not your loved one, but you)? 1. Help me declutter and organize our home. 2. Stay in the house with Herb so I can go to my daughter's baby shower without having to worry about things here at home. 3. Help me find the resources we need. I'm not much good at that. I don't know where to turn.

When was the last time you cried? A few tears leak every day...when he chuckles at my driving or reacts to our little granddaughter...but let it all loose, sob it out, cry? Maybe once or twice when I was in the shower and no one could see when first diagnosed. For now, I have to stay strong for myself and for him. There will be plenty of time for tears later.

Do you like yourself? Usually...but not when I lose my patience and get angry. I sometimes have to remind myself that it's FTD and not my sweet Herb. I forget for a few seconds and get angry at myself for it.

What is the hardest thing you have faced? That there is nothing that can be done for Herb. We can't stop it and he'll never get better.

What is the one thing that no one can understand about your situation? That he can't help how he is or change how he behaves.

What is it that everyone should know, but no one wants to talk about? My family has been behind us...they are there for me to talk to, and if they don't understand something, they ask me. My Herb's family doesn't call to find out how he's doing. They don't seem to want to talk about it. The rare times I talk to his older son and his wife who live out of state, they seem critical. His younger son who lives twenty minutes away never calls or visits, and when they came by for Christmas dinner, not a one of the family so much as went back to our room to say hello. I need to keep in mind that everyone handles grief differently...but Herb is very much still here and needs their love. It's so hard not to get angry.

Do you have support from family? Friends? Church? Others? My family has been great, helping us in any way they can. Other than that, we're pretty much on our own.

What do you miss the most? I miss my best friend and all the fun we used to have camping and doing things with the grandkids. I love the man he is unconditionally but miss terribly the man he was.

Do you have a humorous story you would like to share? Herb kisses me and says he loves me at least a hundred times a day...but even more so at night when we go to bed. He turns in hours before I do, and he struggles to tell me to wake him up when I get there so he can kick me goodnight. He doesn't have a lot of words left and often confuses them in comical ways...so it's become a ritual for me to get my kick goodnight. You need to find the humor where you can...otherwise, the tears can drown you.

Anything else you would like to add? To those who are new to this...be strong and seek help when and where you can. Remember that your mental health matters also.

List any resources that you have found helpful in your journey.

The support groups online are great...the FTD one, the PPA one, and the spouse's group.

ANONYMOUS
Canada

"You have to adapt to accept what you have."

Caree and age at diagnosis: Spouse, 52
Diagnosis: bvFTD, 2016

Where do you find hope? Comfort? I don't have hope, but comfort in family and work.

What is one thing about caregiving (or you or others) that surprised you most? How much I hate it!

How do you take care of yourself? Working incessantly and caring for my farm keeps me exhausted and out of the house, which keeps me sane.

What do you do when you hit bottom? Cry, swear, and listen to loud music.

What is the best/worst thing you have learned about yourself? I am not cut out to be a caregiver, I cannot love my husband as he is now.

What would you most like to tell someone who has become a caregiver? Run!

What would you do if someone handed you $100,000? Run!

What would you do with three extra hours a day? Get my chores done!

What do you wish you had more of? Time.

What are some easy things you do to relax or find joy? Joy? What's that? Sleep and hide from my husband.

What is the best/worst question you have ever been asked? "Is he getting better now?"

What are three things someone could do to help YOU (not your loved one, but you)? A few decent nights out, take over my chores for a week and make mad, passionate love as often as possible.

When was the last time you cried? A couple of weeks ago.

Do you like yourself? Sometimes.

What is the hardest thing you have faced? The fact that the man I loved doesn't give a tin shit whether I live or die.

What is the one thing that no one can understand about your situation? The fact that just because he looks like my husband doesn't make me love him.

What is it that everyone should know, but no one wants to talk about? He is going to die.

Do you have support from family? Friends? Church? Others? Some from friends and family, but they are all far away. Wouldn't touch a church with a very long pole.

What do you miss the most? The new life we planned in Canada.

Anything else you would like to add? Don't try to perpetuate the life you had together before, the person you loved is gone, and trying to pretend they have any of their old feelings will just leave you miserable and disappointed. You have to adapt to accept what you have, because what you had is gone.

List any resources that you have found helpful in your journey. RESPITE!!!

ANONYMOUS
Kansas

"I still grieve my losses every day…"

Caree and age at diagnosis: Spouse, 72
Diagnosis: Frontal lobe syndrome, possibly psychiatric issue, October 2017; TBI, 2004 and 2012; Symptoms of FTD, after 2012.

Where do you find hope? Comfort? God's word, children, caregivers.

What is one thing about caregiving (or you or others) that surprised you most? I was 25+ years caregiver for my son's mental illness and had many crises, one after another. My then husband left, with help from others, was scammed and our retirement was gone. When this happened, I was desperate to stop him, I was actually stunned I couldn't talk him out of it, I surprised myself when I realized, "I can handle this, too!"

How do you take care of yourself? Workouts, devotionals, doing things with my daughter. Husband is still functioning and can be left with someone here. Also, seeing my grandkids and great grandkids.

What do you do when you hit bottom? Happened a lot more with my son. Couldn't get away. Now I stay away from my husband until I can be calm and patient.

What is the best/worst piece of advice you have ever been given? Best: You can't take care of anyone else if you don't take care of yourself first. The brain controls the body, not the other way around. Worst: (about my son), "I'll have him better in 2 weeks!!!"

What is the best/worst thing you have learned about yourself? Best: I am stronger/more understanding. Worst: I cannot contain my emotions without medication most days!

What would you most like to tell someone who has become a caregiver? Find time, even if only 5 minutes, to care for you; don't hesitate to get help from a therapist, etc., journal, whatever it takes to find some calm and peace, if only for a short time.

What would you do if someone handed you $100,000? Half would go into my son's special needs trust. The other half invested until needed for care or an emergency.

What would you do with three extra hours a day? Hang out with my grandchildren and great-grandchildren and daughter, just doing fun stuff and enjoying their company.

What do you wish you had more of? Money now! Our retirement is gone because of other people. It would make me feel less stressed knowing it was there!

What are some easy things you do to relax or find joy? Watch favorite TV shows, read, journal, watch the children, workout, then rest.

What is the best/worst question you have ever been asked? "Do you ever just sit and do nothing?" "Don't you think you're co-dependent?" Arrrrgh.

What are three things someone could do to help YOU (not your loved one, but you)? Household maintenance, yard maintenance, companionship.

When was the last time you cried? A few days ago, mostly depressed and PTSD.

Do you like yourself? Yes! I've done and am doing the best I can in these circumstances.

What is the hardest thing you have faced? No support - emotionally, physically - until last 2 years.

What is the one thing that no one can understand about your situation? How hard it's been on me.

What is it that everyone should know, but no one wants to talk about? I am the expert about my LO's impairment. Almost no one will listen.

Do you have support from family? Friends? Church? Others? Some family, some friends, caregiver's websites.

What do you miss the most? His companionship.

Do you have a humorous story you would like to share? Not at this time.

Anything else you would like to add? I'm grateful for all that I do have and the people in my life right now. I still grieve my losses every day….

List any resources that you have found helpful in your journey.

The right therapist, psychiatrist, journaling, and now caregiver websites.

KATHY
Greenville, NC

"I can learn a lot of things well."

Caree and age at diagnosis: David, 64
Diagnosis: Primary Progressive Aphasia, August 2014

Where do you find hope? Comfort? My primary source of hope is my faith. From the time of diagnosis until now I have turned to my Bible and to music that brings my thoughts and prayers to God. He has been dependably there for me relieving anxiety and guiding me.

What is one thing about caregiving (or you or others) that surprised you most? It has surprised me how many responsibilities that I have acquired and how much others expect of me. But it has also surprised me how well I am doing at my new "job".

How do you take care of yourself? I walk both alone in our neighborhood and also with my LO. Recently, I rediscovered my love of being in the water and joined a deep-water aerobics class which is a great healer of my anxiety and stress. Individual therapy has also gotten me through the years. Friends care about me and my LO, but don't always have the time to listen to me.

What do you do when you hit bottom? Cry and ponder my future. Pray and read spiritually inspiring devotions. Kick myself in the rear and ask for help. Take a nap.

What is the best/worst piece of advice you have ever been given? Best: "Don't expect anything from others, then you won't be disappointed." Worst: "Don't expect to keep him at home. You will need to place him so that you don't go downhill."

What is the best/worst thing you have learned about yourself? Best: That I can learn a lot of things well by asking questions and practicing (financial planning, consulting and planning with building contractors, coordinating my husband's medical needs between providers). Worst: That my emotions can really interfere with my decision making, causing me to decide impulsively for a short-term decision rather than analyze for the long term.

What would you most like to tell someone who has become a caregiver? One of the most important things that has helped me has been to work hard at developing an attitude of being grateful. While this may seem like a spiritual endeavor (as it was for me), it also refers to focusing on the positives in your life that support you in maintaining your physical and mental wellness. The process of focusing on the positives rather than everything that's going wrong has been healing and saved me from being continually stressed out. Writing my thoughts on gratitude into a journal was helpful to the process.

What would you do if someone handed you $100,000? Pay off some of my debt (mortgage, car, etc.) and donate to research on FTD.

What would you do with three extra hours a day? Swim more often, volunteer at church more regularly, and get out and away from my house.

What do you wish you had more of? Contact with my extended family. They live 5-8 hours away.

What are some easy things you do to relax or find joy? Deep breathing. Reading novels that take me away. Prayers of thankfulness. Stroke my super soft little dog, Harry. Cooking (sometimes).

What is the best/worst question you have ever been asked? Best: "Can you come down to stay with us at the beach for a week or whatever number of days work for you?" Worst: "Did David tell you….?" (No, he can't speak.)

What are three things someone could do to help YOU (not your loved one, but you)? Come to stay with him for a few hours to learn about his communication and behavior needs. (That would be a gift to me, too.) Then stay over for a week so that I can go away. Home repairs and advice or work in the yard.

When was the last time you cried? Yesterday.

Do you like yourself? I love myself!

What is the hardest thing you have faced? The change in my relationship with my husband because of his inability to communicate.

What is the one thing that no one can understand about your situation? How important it is to communicate with me. I value conversation and time with others more than anything.

What is it that everyone should know, but no one wants to talk about? That my husband will die from side effects of this horrible disease. Most likely that he will not be able to swallow at all or will aspirate food/liquids into his lungs and we will have to make choices to not resuscitate or to refuse treatment that would prolong his life.

Do you have support from family? Friends? Church? Others? Yes, I have a lot of support from our son who lives in town. Our daughter lives an hour away and is in touch frequently. Friends have offered to help. Extended family have visited periodically, but much less than I thought they would. Church support is awesome and there is more on the horizon. My neighbors are helpful in being my eyes when he is outside or needs help otherwise. I need to be better at asking others to help. I am just discovering how to communicate what I need, and that people really want to know.

What do you miss the most? I miss laughing and talking with him about little things. He doesn't want to do many activities anymore. He can't talk about anything or process what I am saying.

Do you have a humorous story you would like to share? When David was diagnosed with Primary Progressive Aphasia, we had never heard of this disease. We were so relieved that it wasn't Alzheimer's' that we laughed and joked all the way home from the neurology appointment. David told me that he cheated and read the answers to the memory questions on the assessment that were on the score sheet upside down on the doctor's lap. We vowed never to forget those five words. Let's see. Hmmm. "Apple, Yellow, Wagon, ..." So, I guess the joke is on us as he would not be able to get the words out now even if he could remember them. But our naivete about PPA/FTD was entertaining for the ride home.

Anything else you would like to add? It is important to express my heartfelt love for this man with whom I have shared my life since 1979. He has inspired our children and me to keep learning, love the diversity of this world, and to recognize the importance of our family bonds. While he can no longer express his love verbally and his emotions are not focused on the people in his world as they were previously, he deserves my patience and attempted understanding. He recently found my wedding rings on the bedside table one morning and brought them to me, placing them on my finger. I said, "Do you want to marry me?" to which he responded with his sweetest smile. I'm sure he was saying, "yes."

List any resources that you have found helpful in your journey. *Jesus Calling* by Sarah Young. AFTD newsletters. Private Facebook groups – PPA Support Group, the FTD Spouse, and Ask the FTD Patients. *What If It's Not Alzheimer's?* by Radin and Radin.

NANCY
Eagan, MN

"Find ways to give yourself breaks."

Caree and age at diagnosis: David, 56
Diagnosis: ALS/FTD, August 21, 2015

Where do you find hope? Comfort? My relationship with God, constantly giving the situation over to Him, focusing on Him. That is how I made it through. My hope is in Him and Him alone. I received a lot of comfort from family and friends. People all over the world were praying for us from August 2015 forward.

What is one thing about caregiving (or you or others) that surprised you most? How draining and frustrating it can be.

How do you take care of yourself? I purposefully and intentionally kept life as normal as possible for me and my two kids. We stayed involved in church and home-schooling activities; we stayed social as well. I went out for coffee on a consistent basis with different friends. I traveled (5 day trips every quarter). I read, knit, read, knit.... I stayed connected with people and refused to let this disease become our everything.

What do you do when you hit bottom? Talk to God. Talk to a friend with skin on. Get out of the house for a few hours.

What is the best/worst piece of advice you have ever been given? I don't remember getting much advice – good or bad. But the platitudes – I hate those. Or any pity. YUCK!!! The platitude I hate the most is, "God never gives you more than you can handle." That is true because I don't believe God goes around dispensing grief and trials. I do believe He ALLOWS trials and more than we can handle quite often as a way to grab our attention, so we drop to our knees and call out to Him.

What is the best/worst thing you have learned about yourself? The Best: That I am strong. With God's help I can handle what comes my way and I can do it with grace and humor. The Worst: That I can be unbelievably selfish and extremely impatient when things don't go my way.

What would you most like to tell someone who has become a caregiver? Look for humor!!! Find ways to give yourself breaks. Treat yourself kindly, especially in your thoughts about your actions and response to the person you are caring for. Get out and be you, even when it feels selfish. Do not let this disease define you. You will get frustrated!

What would you do if someone handed you $100,000? Bless someone with a portion and invest the rest.

What would you do with three extra hours a day? Read, knit, go out with friends.

What do you wish you had more of? Time with my sister, Lynn. She was my best friend, my person, my other half. We had big plans for after my husband died, then she ended up dying ten weeks after him.

What are some easy things you do to relax or find joy? Read. Knit. Get a massage. Coffee with my friends. Make myself iced coffee.

What is the best/worst question you have ever been asked? No idea.

What are three things someone could do to help YOU (not your loved one, but you)? Bring dinner. Fold loads of clean laundry. Invite me out for coffee. I was blessed on a regular basis with all those things while dealing with being a caregiver.

When was the last time you cried? Yesterday, I was having coffee with a friend and talking about my sister.

Do you like yourself? Yeah, I really do. I also know myself very well. I am very friendly, funny, easy-going, kind, helpful, and transparent. Oh yeah, I can also be selfish and impatient when things don't go the way I want.

What is the hardest thing you have faced? 1. Well the marriage without a diagnosis was extremely hard as there was a lot of nasty behavior to deal with over many years. 2. Telling my kids that their dad had a terminal illness and only 6-24 months to live. They were 14 and 11 at the time. 3. But hands down…losing my sister. As I stated above, she was my person. We just got each other. We talked multiple times in a day. I flew my other sister and myself down to Florida to be with her at the end. She was barely recognizable, so ravaged by cancer. 36 hours after arriving we were told to evacuate because of Hurricane Irma. I kept the rental car and drove home to Minnesota (3 days). My sister died the day after I got home. My brother-in-law didn't have the courage to tell me she was gone so, I found out hours after everyone else and from HIS sister. Weird. But it doesn't matter much. Her being gone is the hardest part. I will miss her to my very marrow all my remaining days.

What is the one thing that no one can understand about your situation? How I could stay so positive, upbeat, and happy and how I could find the humor in the hard things.

What is it that everyone should know, but no one wants to talk about? How incredibly challenging it is to deal with behavioral disorders, especially in adults; how financially draining this illness can be; how screwed up the healthcare system is in America.

Do you have support from family? Friends? Church? Others? Yes. All of the above, as well as an incredible hospice team and FB friends.

What do you miss the most? Having a spouse to talk to about what is happening in life. Physical intimacy.

Do you have a humorous story you would like to share? One day our Pastor of Adult Ministry came for breakfast and to serve us communion. As soon as we finished, and he had prayed. My husband raises his head and announces, "I think I need to go poop!" Oh boy! Talk about embarrassing. Just then the pastor says, "For what it's worth Nance, I'll probably have to go poop later on today, too." I laughed, and the situation was diffused.

Anything else you would like to add? Nope.

List any resources that you have found helpful in your journey. Holy Bible. *Jesus Calling* by Sarah Young. The FTD Spouse Facebook page. The AFTD with Children in the Home monthly support call.

MY STORY

(your name here)

(your city and state)

(your quote)

Caree and age at diagnosis:

Diagnosis:

    Where do you find hope? Comfort?

    What is one thing about caregiving (or you or others) that surprised you most?

    How do you take care of yourself?

    What do you do when you hit bottom?

    What is the best/worst piece of advice you have ever been given?

What is the best/worst thing you have learned about yourself?

What would you most like to tell someone who has become a caregiver?

What would you do if someone handed you $100,000?

What would you do with three extra hours a day?

What do you wish you had more of?

What are some easy things you do to relax or find joy?

What is the best/worst question you have ever been asked?

What are three things someone could do to help YOU (not your loved one, but you)?

When was the last time you cried?

Do you like yourself?

What is the hardest thing you have faced?

What is the one thing that no one can understand about your situation?

What is it that everyone should know, but no one wants to talk about?

Do you have support from family? Friends? Church? Others?

What do you miss the most?

Do you have a humorous story you would like to share?

Anything else you would like to add?

List any resources that you have found helpful in your journey.

ACKNOWLEDGMENTS

First and foremost, this book would not have been possible without the caregivers who were willing to share their stories. Their willingness to share their hopes, fears, joys, and struggles is a testament to their bravery. Sharon Hall, one of the interviewees, calls the FTD caregiving community her "redwoods". Redwood trees are impressive in size, but their real strength comes from their intertwining root system. Each redwood helps to hold up its neighboring redwoods. By standing together, holding roots, they are able to withstand the elements that would bring them down. In a similar manner, the caregiving community strengthens its members by taking turns leaning on each other and sharing strength. Without this community, this journey would be overwhelming.

I am indebted to my friends, Beth Ruehrdanz and Marlene Mahn, who read the initial manuscript and found the grammatical and punctuation errors.

Finally, I want to thank my Stephen minister, Karen Stiehl, and my dear friends, Diana Vander Pas, Liesl James, Pam Willmann, Dawn Lange, and Rachel Morton. These ladies constantly encourage me, listen to me cry, pray for me, and remind me that God can, and will, use this experience to his glory.

APPENDIX 1: SUGGESTED READING

Boss, Pauline. *Loving Someone Who Has Dementia.* San Francisco, CA: Jossey-Bass, 2011.

-*Ambiguous Loss: Learning to Live with Unresolved Grief.* Cambridge, MA: Harvard University Press, 2000.

Dunlop, John. *Finding Grace in the Face of Dementia.* Wheaton, IL: Crossway, 2017.

Guthrie, Nancy. *One Year Book of Hope.* Carol Stream, IL: Tyndale House Publishers, 2005.

Hone, Lucy. *Resilient Grieving: Finding Strength and Embracing Life After a Loss That Changes Everything.* New York, NY: The Experiment, 2017.

Mace, Nancy L. and Peter V. Rabins. *The 36 Hour Day.* Baltimore, MD: John Hopkins University Press, 2017.

Neff, Kristin. *Self-Compassion: The Proven Power of Being Kind to Yourself.* New York, NY: Harper Collins Publications, 2015.

Radin, Gary and Lisa Radin. *What If It's Not Alzheimer's.* Amherst, NY: Prometheus Books, 2014.

Toth, Susan Allen. *No Saints Around Here.* Minneapolis, MN: University of Minnesota Press, 2014.

Williams, Marie. *Green Vanilla Tea.* Oakland, CA: New Harbinger Publications, Inc., 2014.

Young, Sarah. *Jesus Calling.* Nashville, TN: Thomas Nelson, 2004.

The Holy Bible: The Book of Psalms

APPENDIX 2: RESOURCES

Alexa – voice activated assistant

Alfred Camera App – app that allows you to use old smartphones with cameras as security cameras for free

The Alzheimer's Association – www.alz.org

Amazon – www.amazon.com

The Association for Frontotemporal Degeneration – www.theaftd.org

Caregiving.com – www.caregiving.com – FTD chat and FTD podcasts

Dementia Care – Love, Laughter, Tears, and Lessons with Gilly B. – on YouTube

The FTD Spouse on Facebook

Google – www.google.com

Grocery Delivery – Shipt – www.shipt.com
　　　　　　　　　　Instacart – www.instacart.com
　　　　　　　(as well as many others)

Grocery Delivery - Curbside – www.clicklist.com – Kroger

Holding Space – www.heatherplett.com/holdingpsace

Mindfulness Meditations – www.mindful.org

National Institute on Aging - www.nia.nih.gov/health/caregiving

RoadId – www.roadid.com – ID bracelets with document storage capability

Teepa Snow – www.teepasnow.com

TSA Cares – www.tsa.gov/travel/passenger-support

YouTube – www.youtube.com

ABOUT THE AUTHOR

Martha Garmon lives in Paris, Texas with her husband, Stephan and her two dogs, Coco and Chewie. She has a son, Brandon, and daughter, Leia. She has a granddaughter and a grandson. Martha has her doctorate in Worship Studies and retired from her position as Minister of Worship and Music at Prince of Peace Lutheran Church in Palatine, Illinois in December 2018. She is also the primary caregiver for her husband Stephan who was diagnosed with frontotemporal degeneration in July 2016 and ALS in February 2018.

Made in the USA
Middletown, DE
20 March 2021